If Foods Could Heal:

Reverse and Prevent Disease, Boost Immunity, and Eat Your Way to Better Health with the Anti-Inflammatory Diet

ERRYN O'CAIN, PharmD

DEDICATION

To my father, Alan, who taught me the value of independent thought, and to my late mother, Charletta, who taught me to love everyone as I love myself.

CONTENTS

Introduction   1

1   What Is Inflammation and Why Is It a Bad   4
    Thing?

2   Understanding the Science   9

3   Symptoms of Chronic Inflammation   25

4   Foods That Trigger Inflammation   40

5   Anti-Inflammatory Foods   49

6   The Anti-Inflammatory Diet   60

7   10 Wholesome Anti-Inflammatory Recipes   70

8   10 Anti-Inflammatory Drinks   92

9   The Anti-Inflammatory Lifestyle   114

10 The Inflammation Spectrum   120

    Final Words   140

    References   142

    About Author   147

INTRODUCTION

You are likely reading this book because you've experienced symptoms of inflammation or are struggling with a health concern. You may be constantly tired, have body aches, recurrent colds, and flu, persisting digestive issues, or you may struggle with your weight.

There is no single solution for every person because, as you'll learn later on, each of our microbiomes at the gut level is unique. Certain foods, exposures, and stress levels may trigger inflammation in one person while not affecting another. What inflammation does in your body is also unique. It may cause weight gain and fatigue in your spouse, acid reflux in a parent, and something entirely different in you.

Where inflammation occurs in your body will be dependent on your genetics, lifestyle, past injuries, and the environment you live in. It tends to develop in eight different areas, and you may have symptoms in many of these to a lesser or greater degree:

Brain and nervous system

Brain fog, depression, anxiety, mood swings, lack of focus, trouble concentrating, poor memory, or a general feeling of malaise.

Digestive tract

Constipation, diarrhea, stomach aches, bloating, and heartburn. You may also experience a distended and swollen stomach due to water retention.

Detoxification processes (liver, kidneys, gallbladder, and lymphatic system)

Waste isn't processed efficiently, and it tends to back up in your system. Your limbs and belly may swell, you could have aches and pains, or you frequently get rashes on your skin.

Blood sugar and insulin balance (liver, pancreas, and cellular insulin receptor sites)

Unstable blood sugar levels, excess insulin, metabolic syndrome, prediabetes, or type 2 diabetes. Symptoms can include excessive hunger and thirst, rapid weight gain or loss, and high blood sugar levels.

Endocrine system (hormone-producing glands such as thyroid, adrenals, ovaries, or testes)

Thinning hair, dry skin, weak nails, anxiety, mood swings, irregular menstruation, or low sex drive. It can also manifest in severe premenstrual syndrome (PMS) symptoms, polycystic ovary syndrome (PCOS), and uterine fibroids.

Musculoskeletal system (muscles, joints, and connective tissue)

Joint pain and stiffness, muscle pain, fibromyalgia (a condition connected to autoimmunity), body aches, and muscular spasms.

Immune system

When your immune system overreacts and attacks your own organs, tissues, or structures of the body, it's called autoimmunity. The autoimmune response can impact every system in the body, including the digestive system (for example, celiac disease or inflammatory bowel disease), the brain and nervous system (multiple sclerosis), the joints and connective tissue (rheumatoid arthritis and lupus), the thyroid gland (Hashimoto's thyroiditis), as well as a multitude of inflammatory skin conditions.

The good news is that all inflammation can be decreased through an intelligent diet, no matter its cause or effect. The goal is to minimize foods that are known to trigger inflammatory responses and eat more foods proven to lower inflammation.

This book will teach how to do exactly that.

1

WHAT IS INFLAMMATION AND WHY IS IT A BAD THING?

Not all inflammation is harmful. Your body needs it to survive, fight disease, and heal. Our immune system is designed to fight microscopic threats and usually does its job exceptionally well. Inflammation is our body's response to danger, and it's the only way we manage to stay healthy. However, there are two types of inflammation - one is good and necessary, and one is harmful and destructive.

Acute Inflammation

Acute inflammation is our body's healing mechanism. If you injure yourself, you'll notice swelling in the area, for example, after spraining your ankle or pulling a muscle. This inflammation may be red and hot, a sign that your body is trying to heal itself, and the pain keeps you from using that part of your body. This is when inflammation is of tremendous benefit.

Chronic Inflammation

Chronic inflammation, when left untreated, can lead to serious long-term complications. This is when the body starts to attack itself (and not an infection or injury). It will continue to do so unless addressed.

Here's what happens with chronic inflammation. Let's say your immune system is trying to fight infections such as Lyme disease but seems to be failing miserably. In this case, your immunity seems to be too busy to be effective. Or, perhaps your immune system gets confused, like a person who has antibodies to gluten that suddenly start attacking any part of the body that resembles gluten.

Chronic inflammation also happens when the immune system picks up that something isn't quite right. For example, when (low-density lipoproteins) LDL cholesterol penetrates the lining of an artery. White blood cells tag along but, instead of helping, they end up making it worse. The plaque becomes unstable and more likely to rupture.

This kind of self-damaging attack happens all around the body in inflamed areas. We'll go into great detail on the symptoms and consequences of inflammation in another chapter but, for now, it will help to know the top five symptoms of chronic inflammation. If this sounds like you, you'll know you need to read further!

Body Pain (muscles and joints)

Muscle aches and joint pain are often caused by inflammation. When defensive cytokines are elevated in the body, they can inadvertently attack muscle and joint tissue. This results in redness, swelling, and pain, despite no obvious injury.

Skin rashes (includes swelling and infection)

Inflammatory skin conditions such as adult acne and skin rashes (eczema or psoriasis) often occur. You may have red, rough, and flaky skin. These skin conditions are linked to hypersensitivity of the immune system, and a rash can be triggered almost instantaneously after eating an inflammatory food.

Excessive mucus production

Suppose you find that you're constantly needing to clear your throat or blow your nose, even when you don't have a cold or allergy. In that case, you're likely suffering from some level of inflammation. When inflamed, mucous membranes produce thick phlegm. They are trying to protect the respiratory system with a protective lining. This buildup results in coughing, sneezing, and a runny nose.

Low energy (including libido)

Despite getting enough sleep, a constant feeling of fatigue and exhaustion is another common symptom. When you're chronically inflamed, your immune system is active (it's literally at war) and works overtime to try and restore balance. This requires a lot more energy from your cells, with continual regeneration of immune cells, all of which deplete you of the fuel you need to stay alert and energized.

Poor digestion (and increased or decreased appetite)

Common inflammatory symptoms with the digestive tract include bloating, abdominal pain, constipation, and loose stool. Chronic inflammation throughout the body also contributes to leaky gut syndrome (intestinal permeability), which can cause bacteria and toxins to "leak" through the intestinal wall into the rest of the body. This can also fuel ongoing inflammation throughout the body and its systems, furthering digestive abnormalities like distension and irregular bowel movements.

Controlling Chronic Inflammation

Most health problems that we struggle with - fatigue, digestive issues, hormone imbalances, diabetes, heart disease, depression, and autoimmune conditions - have an inflammatory component.

The problem with inflammation is that we often don't even notice it is happening until we experience advanced symptoms. Inflammation may have done incredible damage to your body before you receive an accurate diagnosis of your illness, oftentimes after a few years of pain, discomfort, and general malaise.

You don't simply wake up one day with diabetes or arthritis. Inflammation was likely brewing for years before. Doctor Will Cole, the author of Inflammation Spectrum, says: "Lifestyle and foods are the primary methods for reducing the inflammation that leads to disease" (Cole, 2021). He goes on to explain that studies estimate around 77 percent of our inflammatory reactions are determined by factors we have control over. This includes our diets, stress levels, and exposure to pollutants. Only 23 percent is due to genetics. This is brilliant news - it means that there is much we can do to reduce inflammation in our bodies and take control of our health.

Before we investigate the types of food and lifestyle choices that impact the inflammatory response in our bodies, however, it's important to understand the science behind how it all works. We'll look at that in the next chapter.

2

UNDERSTANDING THE SCIENCE

Your body's immune response and inflammation all start in your digestive tract. It's important to understand how bacteria functions in your gut, how this is essential for your survival, and how eating the incorrect types of food can throw the entire system out of whack.

Let's start with getting to know the sensitive and complicated world of bacteria in your intestines.

The Gut Microbiome

Our gut contains around 100 trillion bacteria. Different types of bacteria produce different substances, such as gases, acids, and fats. They help us process food, supply energy, convert and manufacture vitamins, break down various toxins and medications, and have a delicate and substantial relationship with the immune system. Our microbiome plays a massive role in how the immune system responds in the body and is responsible for much of the balance - and imbalance - of inflammation. When something is out of sorts with our microbiome, our entire body feels it.

The bulk of our immune system (around 80 percent) is found in the gut. Each of us has a unique microbial landscape, and our different types of bacteria respond in different ways to food, medicine, toxins, and viruses. What triggers an inflammatory response in one person after eating a sandwich will be harmless for another person. Although there are obvious commonalities, much of living an anti-inflammatory lifestyle is a game of trial and error and getting to know your own individual microbiome and how it reacts to certain foods.

Despite the incredible diversity of our bacterial constitutions, there are two basic gut types, and you'll likely recognize yourself as dominant in one of them. Your specific microbe make-up depends on which family of bacteria dominate your digestive tract: Bacteroides or Prevotella. These families of bacteria break down food in different ways, produce different types of molecules and proteins, and will attack certain harmful substances while choosing to leave others alone. They can also change the terrain of the microbiome by how they interact with the other two groups of bacteria. There may be a friendly relationship, or they may go all-out and attack anything that doesn't look like themself.

Let's take a closer look at the two different gut types:

Gut Type One: Bacteroides
These are usually the most prevalent in the gut and are the kings of breaking down carbohydrates, proteins, and fiber.

They generate the precise enzymes they need for almost anything that travels through your gut, and they are very good at extracting energy from food that passes through. They have a particular preference for meat and saturated fatty acids, and they abound in the guts of people who eat a lot of animal products. As this type of bacteria is also good at pulling energy from food, the people who have this group dominating their system tend to struggle with rapid weight gain (and struggle to lose weight too).

This group of bacteria is also very proficient at producing large amounts of biotin (vitamin B7 and H). Biotin promotes healthy-looking skin, shiny hair, and strong nails and is also involved in other vital processes such as synthesizing carbs and fats.

You'll pick up that you have a biotin deficiency if you have brittle hair and nails, are lethargic, experience increased infections, and have higher levels of cholesterol in your blood. Antibiotics are known to cause biotin deficiency.

Gut Type Two: Prevotella

The dominance of this group of bacteria is most common in vegetarians. This bacterium produces vitamin B1 (thiamine), which is largely responsible for our nerve and brain health. A thiamine deficiency can result in muscle tremors and memory loss. It's also responsible for irritability, frequent headaches, and decreased concentration.

Understanding Prebiotics

You are now more aware of the importance of probiotics. In summary, they are essential for digestion and help the microbiome in your gut stay healthy. They are usually found in yogurt, fermented products, and supplements. The probiotics in your colon improve your health on all levels - physically, mentally, and emotionally. They increase the absorption of minerals, strengthen your bowel wall, and help regulate hormone production.

Prebiotics are not as well-known and are basically the probiotics' food. Prebiotics, a type of plant fiber, provide nutrients to the good bacteria in your gastrointestinal tract. Probiotics, as you now know, vary from person to person. Different people have different reactions, so it's difficult to know which type of probiotic is the best type for each individual. This is what makes prebiotics so powerful.

Prebiotics, on their own, may help with weight loss, reduce inflammation and inflammatory bowel disease, help to prevent certain cancers (such as colon and rectal cancer), lower your risk for cardiovascular disease, and enhance calcium absorption. They are also effective at treating diarrhea, preventing yeast infections, and reduce the severity of illnesses like the common cold. Prebiotics and probiotics are both good at lowering cholesterol.

Prebiotics may also have a direct influence on mental health. In 2013, Neurochemistry International observed that prebiotics increase brain-derived neurotrophic factor (BDNF) expression. Although more studies and research still need to be done, it's a promising indicator that prebiotics can be used to help treat neuropsychiatric illnesses, such as Alzheimer's and depression, and can also improve memory and concentration (Laboratories, n.d.). In addition, they may lower your risk of heart disease because they improve the function of the lining of your blood vessels, arteries, and capillaries.

All prebiotics are made of fiber, but not all fibers are

considered prebiotic. The plant fiber needs to be fermented by the intestinal microflora, stimulate the growth and activity of good bacteria, be resistant to gastric activity, and be absorbed in the upper gastrointestinal tract to qualify as a prebiotic.

Prebiotics are found naturally in fiber-rich foods such as asparagus, chicory, leeks, artichokes, wheat, soybeans, oats, garlic, and onions. They're also in apple skins, so don't peel those before you eat them.

Prebiotics and probiotics work in synergy, and it's important to have both of them in your diet.

The Body's Immune Response

The immune response is your body's way of recognizing and defending itself against bacteria, viruses, and other foreign and harmful substances. It does this by responding to antigens. Antigens can be proteins found on the surface of cells (your own body's or fungi, for instance) and also consist of non-living substances such as toxins, drugs, and foreign particles (such as a thorn in your foot). The immune system tries to destroy substances that contain antigens.

Some of your body's cells have human leukocyte antigens (HLA) on their surface. These proteins are recognized by your immune system but seen as normal, and usually, there is no reaction to them.

It's important to understand the different types of immune responses to understand why your body's immunity causes inflammation.

Innate Immunity
This is the defense system you are born with and protects

you against all antigens. It keeps harmful substances from entering your body and is the first line of defense. This includes things like the cough reflex, enzymes in tears, mucus that traps bacteria, stomach acid, and the skin barrier.

There are also protein chemical forms of innate immunity and include substances, such as interferon and interleukin-1, that cause pain and fever.

If an antigen manages to get past these initial barriers, it is attacked by other parts of the immune system.

Acquired Immunity

This line of defense develops after exposure to specific antigens. Your body recognizes and destroys them immediately. This is why if you had measles once, you'll likely never have it again. You are now immune to that particular virus.

Passive Immunity

When antibodies are produced in your body that isn't your own, it's called passive immunity. Newborns have passive immunity because they received their antibodies through the placenta from their mothers. You can also receive this defense when you are injected with an antiserum containing antibodies formed by another person or animal. You'll have immediate protection against a particular antigen, but it doesn't last forever. For example, you have passive immunity after getting a shot for hepatitis exposure or tetanus.

Immunization

Vaccinations trigger the body's immune response. Small doses of an antigen, usually a weak form of a live virus, are injected to activate the immune system's 'memory,' which includes activated B cells and sensitized T cells. This triggers your body to react quickly to future exposures. For example, getting a Covid-19 vaccination allows your body to attack exposure to the virus by responding much faster and more effectively to the presence of these antigens in your body.

Immunity in Your Blood

One of your immune system's primary defense mechanisms is white blood cells, assisted by chemicals, antibodies, other proteins, and interferon. Some immediately attack foreign substances, and others work in a team to assist the immune response.

White blood cells include B and T lymphocytes, and they are your body's powerful line of defense.

B lymphocytes turn into cells that produce antibodies that attach to a specific antigen. This makes it easier for other immune cells to destroy the antigen. It's just like a soldier immobilizing an enemy then sending up a flare to call in the troops.

T lymphocytes attack antigens directly. They also release chemicals called cytokines that control the entire immune response.

Lymphocytes usually tell the difference between your own body tissues and foreign antigens very well. They multiply and provide 'memory' for your immune system, which allows your body to respond faster when you're exposed to the same antigen, and you often won't even know about it because you won't get sick at all (despite having just fought off a virus in your body). This is the acquired immunity we mentioned earlier.

When Immunity Goes Wrong

Problems with the immune system occur when the immune response is targeted against your body's own tissue, when it "over-responds," or when it doesn't respond at all. Allergies, for example, are an immune response to a harmless substance, such as peanuts.

An immune system that is overactive can lead to autoimmune diseases, and the body forms antibodies against its own tissues.

Inflammation and Immunity

When tissues are injured by bacteria, trauma, or toxins, the body responds through inflammation. If you burn your hand, for example, the damaged cells release chemicals alerting your body that you are hurt. These chemicals cause your blood vessels to leak fluid into the tissue resulting in swelling. They also attract a type of white blood cell, known as phagocytes, to the area. These absorb the germs and dead or damaged cells and eventually die themselves. When this defensive process happens, you'll notice pus form in the area - it's a collection of dead tissue, bacteria, and phagocytes.

Inflammation, in most cases, is a positive thing, but it can also go very wrong.

Acute and Chronic Inflammation

Infections, wounds, and tissue damage would not be able to heal without our body's inflammatory response. There are two types of inflammation: acute and chronic.

Acute Inflammation: This happens very quickly and usually resolves on its own in under two weeks. Your body responds to the injury or toxin, repairs damaged cells and removes dead cells. Common symptoms include redness, swelling, heat, and pain. You'll have experienced this type of inflammation every time you've had a sore throat, pimple, or ingrown toenail. It's also there when you sprain your ankle, forcing you to not put any weight on that leg and protecting your body against further injury.

Chronic Inflammation: This is a slower and less noticeable form of inflammation. Sometimes your body isn't able to remove the harmful substance or effectively heal an injury. The body can remain inflamed for years. It may also occur if the toxin has been eliminated, but the body still stays in a state of inflammation.

This chronic and ongoing inflammation has the following symptoms: body pain, constant fatigue, depression, anxiety, digestion problems (such as pain, constipation, diarrhea, and bloating), weight fluctuation, and frequent infections (such as urinary tract infections).

If you have chronic inflammation, you will know and feel that something isn't quite right. You feel unwell and exhausted, get sick often, your stomach gives you problems, and your brain might feel foggy. This general sense of being under the weather for no reason, for an extended period of time, is most often due to chronic inflammation.

How the Inflammatory Flame Is Stoked

Apart from diet, which we will be looking at in great detail in this book, there are other contributing factors that fuel inflammation:

- Being overweight or obese

- High levels of stress
- Irregular sleep and insomnia
- Smoking, alcohol, and drug abuse
- Age, Perimenopause, and Menopause
- Polluted environments and products
- Allergies, Sensitivities, and Intolerances

There are certain foods and food products that you may need to avoid because your body has a specific response to them.

Food Allergies

This is caused by an overreaction of the immune system to a particular food or beverage. They tend to show symptoms immediately and can range from a tiny rash and watery eyes to swelling and anaphylactic shock. Common allergies include shellfish and peanuts.

Food Sensitivities

These are often delayed, more chronic symptoms. It can exhibit as fatigue, nasal congestion, or joint pain - even several days after eating a specific food. Food sensitivities are usually caused by nutrient deficiencies or by eating too much of one type of food day after day.

If you have a food sensitivity, it doesn't mean you necessarily have to eliminate the food types and never enjoy them again. As you'll soon see, there are many foods that can cause a reaction and it's impossible to remove them all from your diet. There are some that are also often recommended in anti-inflammatory diets.

In the last chapter, we'll go in-depth around the topic of

bio-individuality. You'll learn that your body is highly unique. You may be sensitive to one histamine food type yet feel nourished with another. You need to find your sweet spot.

You'll know when you've eaten something and your body feels a little off afterward. The sensitivity lists are simply here to guide you, making you aware of potential sensitivities, and then it's up to you to determine your unique reactions and what you personally need to avoid.

Sensitivity to Histamines

Histamines are produced by your immune system to defend your body against allergens. If too much is released, or if they are triggered when it isn't necessary, they can cause various symptoms. This can range from normal allergy symptoms, such as an itchy throat and stuffy nose, to skin rashes, digestive problems, joint pain, and neurological symptoms.

People with a sensitivity to histamines may notice these kinds of symptoms after eating cured meat, fermented foods, or wine. Gastrointestinal tract issues, such as small intestinal bacterial overgrowth (SIBO), are often the cause of histamine intolerance. Sometimes addressing this helps resolve the sensitivity to histamine.

If you're particularly responsive to histamine and your body is showing adverse reactions, try to cut down on foods that are naturally high in histamine. They may trigger an overloaded response which leads to inflammation. These high-histamine foods include:

- Alcohol (especially wine and beer)
- Bone broth
- Canned food
- Cheese (especially mature cheese)

- Chocolate
- Eggplant
- Fermented foods (such as kefir, kimchi, yogurt, and sauerkraut)
- Legumes (most particularly fermented soybeans, chickpeas, and peanuts)
- Mushrooms
- Nuts (especially cashews and walnuts)
- Processed foods
- Shellfish
- Smoked meat (such as bacon, salami, salmon, and ham)
- Spinach
- Vinegar

The following foods, while low in histamines themselves, can trigger their release. If you're intolerant to histamine, it will help to cut down on the following:

- Avocados
- Bananas
- Citrus fruits (for example, lemons, limes, oranges, and grapefruit)
- Strawberries
- Tomatoes

Diamine Oxidase (DAO) Enzyme Blockers

These foods block the enzyme that controls histamine. They can result in higher levels in some people:

- Alcohol
- Energy drinks

- Teas (black, green, yerba mate)

Sensitivity to Salicylates

These compounds are found in pain medications such as aspirin. They're also hidden in beauty and skincare products. When it comes to diet, they occur naturally in certain plant foods.

Symptoms of salicylate intolerance are similar to those of histamine and include neurological, digestive, and skin reactions. The following foods are salicylate-rich:

- Almonds
- Apricots
- Avocados
- Blackberries
- Cherries
- Coconut oil
- Dates
- Dried fruits
- Endive
- Gherkins
- Grapes
- Green olives
- Guavas
- Honey
- Nightshades (these include peppers, eggplant, tomatoes, and potatoes)
- Olive oil
- Oranges
- Pineapple

- Plums and prunes
- Tangelos
- Tangerines
- Water chestnuts

Sensitivity to FODMAPs

Some people experience gastrointestinal symptoms when they eat high-fructose fruits and certain vegetables, legumes, sweeteners, and wheat. This is usually indicative of a sensitivity to fermentable oligosaccharides, disaccharides, monosaccharides, and polyols (which are all much more widely known as FODMAPs).

This group of carbohydrate foods can cause IBS-type symptoms such as constipation, diarrhea, stomach cramps, and bloating. Some people are tolerant of many FODMAP foods but react to others. You may need to eliminate and reintroduce FODMAP foods one at a time and see how your body reacts. FODMAP foods include:

- Artichoke
- Asparagus
- Bananas
- Beets
- Cabbage
- Cashews
- Carob powder
- Cauliflower
- Coconut water
- Dairy products (derived specifically from cows milk - cheese, milk, cream, ice-cream, sour cream, and yogurt)

- Fruit juice
- Garlic
- Gluten (any products that contain wheat, barley, rye, or spelt)
- Green beans
- High-fructose fruits (that's all of them except berries, limes, lemons, and melons)
- Honey
- Legumes
- Mushrooms
- Onions (all types, including shallots and scallions)
- Peas
- Sauerkraut
- Soy
- Sugar alcohols (these are often used in sugar-free sweets: inulin, isomalt, maltitol, mannitol, sorbitol, xylitol)

Sensitivity to Oxalates

Oxalates bind to minerals to form calcium oxalate and iron oxalate. This can take place in the digestive tract, kidneys, or urinary tract, driving inflammation in these areas. Cooking veggies will lower their oxalate levels.

If you're sensitive to oxalates, these are the foods you need to be cautious of:

- Beets
- Cocoa
- Kale
- Peanuts

- Spinach
- Sweet potatoes
- Swiss chard

Food Intolerance

This is when your system lacks a compound that is essential for digesting a certain type of food. For instance, if you are lacking lactase (the enzyme that breaks down lactose), you may be intolerant of milk and dairy products. Symptoms can include cramping, diarrhea, or bloating. All of these food reactions can also lead directly to inflammation.

Inflammation may be an underlying cause of multiple diseases. For example, the leaky gut syndrome is a part of the mechanism in which food allergies, sensitivities, intolerances, and toxins trigger autoimmune diseases.

Autoimmune diseases are chronic diseases in which the body attacks itself with inflammation that is completely out of control. Dietary factors play an important role in autoimmunity. For example, people with Sjögren's disease and Graves' disease have a greater intolerance to gluten and a higher risk of developing celiac disease.

In the next chapter, we will take a closer look at what chronic inflammation looks like in the body, what the symptoms are, and the effect of letting inflammation go unaddressed for too long.

3

SYMPTOMS OF CHRONIC INFLAMMATION

Many things contribute to chronic inflammation. Some triggers you can't help, such as your genetic predisposition. However, most you have control over, including your sleep patterns and, very importantly, your diet.

Let's have a look at what chronic inflammation looks like in the body.

Symptoms of Chronic Inflammation

- Blocked or runny nose - Inflamed nasal cavities is one way your body tries to protect itself against foreign substances or infection, such as with a common cold or allergies. However, if your nose is consistently like this, it can be a sign of chronic inflammation.

- Weight gain or weight loss - Chronic inflammation can increase your metabolism, which may lead to weight loss. It can also interfere with your body's response to a hormone called leptin which is what lets your brain know you've had enough to eat. Without this signal, we tend to overindulge and gain weight.

- Your memory and concentration may be affected by inflammation, which also has a role to play in depression, anxiety, and mood disorders. In older people, inflammation can contribute to Alzheimer's disease and dementia. You may simply feel as if your thinking is not as clear as it once was. Concentration becomes difficult, and you may start forgetting simple things like appointments.

- You may struggle with your balance. Some chronic inflammatory diseases (CIDs) cause your body to react aggressively, sometimes attacking itself in the process. In one such disease, multiple sclerosis, the body's immune system attacks the myelin sheath of the nerves (their insulation coating). This makes it more difficult for nerve signals to be transmitted, and you may feel dizzy and off-balance.

- Insulin resistance - Although this doesn't always exhibit symptoms, inflammation can affect how well the insulin in your body works. Insulin helps control your blood sugar levels, and when you're insulin resistant, your blood sugar spikes. This, in turn, damages your nerves and blood vessels and can lead to diabetes. Your hands and feet may tingle due to poor circulation, and you may be thirstier and more fatigued than normal.

- Muscle weakening - When your immune system attacks your muscles and causes inflammation, it's called myositis. Muscle fibers get broken down, and this can lead to weakness. It often starts slowly but can become debilitating as it can affect your ability to do simple activities such as walking and swallowing.

- Digestive issues such as gassiness, constipation, diarrhea, bloating, and cramping - Inflammatory bowel disease (IBD) usually expresses itself in two forms: ulcerative colitis and Crohn's disease. Both of these are caused by inflammation of the colon and small intestine. Symptoms include diarrhea, nausea, joint pain, fever, and skin rashes. Irritable bowel syndrome (IBS) and food allergies are often due to inflammation, as are heartburn and gastric acid reflux.

- Lower back pain and stiffness, especially in the morning - This occurs when chronic inflammation attacks the spine and is called ankylosing spondylitis. It can also affect your hips, neck, knees, and chest.

- Constant fatigue - One of the most common symptoms of inflammation and inflammatory diseases such as fibromyalgia, multiple sclerosis, lupus, and rheumatoid arthritis. Always feeling tired with constant drops in energy is often indicative of inflammation. It can also lead to insomnia and other sleep issues such as trouble falling asleep, constant waking, restless tossing and turning, and waking up exhausted.

- Too much or too little sleep can cause inflammation. The cells in your body respond to this irregularity as if it were an illness. It also becomes a vicious cycle because inflammation causes sleeping disturbances.

- Skin breakouts and rashes - Very often, what is going on inside of our bodies also happens on the outside. When it comes to inflammation, it can develop as a rash, acne, dry skin, and eczema.

- Livedo reticularis rash - This is a purple, marbled-looking rash that usually occurs on your arms and legs and is often present with inflammatory conditions such as lupus and antiphospholipid syndrome. It's more noticeable when it's cold and sometimes goes away on its own.

- Arteriosclerosis or hardening of the arteries - This is when there is fatty plaque buildup on the inner walls of your arteries and can lead to heart attack and stroke. This fat residue is the body's inflammatory response to high body fat and also toxic substances, such as cigarette smoke.

- Dry eyes are another common symptom of inflammation. This can feel like a gritty sensation, and some people complain of burning, sore eyes. One particular condition called Sjögren's syndrome attacks your salivary and tear glands. This shows up as swollen salivary glands and a dry nose and throat.

- Abnormal blood clotting (hypercoagulation) can be caused by inflammation due to trauma or injury, surgery, or diseases like inflammatory bowel disease (IBD). It can cause swelling and even more serious problems such as a stroke or heart attack.

- Body pain, arthralgia (joint pain), and myalgia (muscle pain) -This also includes nerve pain, general aches, and spasms.

- Frequent infections - Everything from urinary tract infections to slow-healing wounds.

- Unexplained aches and pains that aren't due to an injury - If you flex and extend your arm, for example, and you feel a twinge at the end of your range of motion (either in your elbow or your muscles), you could have inflammation.

- Swollen lymph nodes - These are located in your neck, armpits, and near the groin. When these are swollen, it's a sign that something is out of balance. Your immune system may be responding to an infection (such as a cold), but it may also be pointing towards chronic inflammation, especially if they are constantly sore and swollen.

- Headaches and/or migraines - Neurogenic inflammation in the brain can cause headaches and is often caused by lifestyle choices such as smoking, alcohol consumption, and stress.

When Things Get Nasty

Chronic inflammation, when left untreated, can result in severe and potentially life-threatening illnesses.

Heart Disease

Clinical research shows a strong connection between inflammation and heart disease, which is the leading cause of death for men and women. Inflammation exacerbates atherosclerosis, the fatty deposits that build up in the lining of our arteries.

If inflammation damages blood vessels, then cholesterol is used to patch them up. This creates plaque that can lead directly to those fatty deposits, as well as other heart-related diseases. These can range from minor arrhythmia to a major heart attack.

Here Are the Usual Heart Inflammation Suspects:

1. Cardiovascular disease (also known as atherosclerosis) is the hardening of the arteries and is caused by the buildup of fatty plaques in the blood vessels. It makes them hard and stiff. This is triggered by lifestyle choices such as smoking, obesity, lack of exercise, and an unhealthy diet.

2. Coronary heart or artery disease - This is when there is plaque buildup in the arteries of the heart itself. More than 500,000 people die from coronary artery disease in the United States alone each year.

3. The buildup of fatty plaque can lead to angina, or chest pain, mainly because the heart isn't receiving enough blood. This can get worse over time and eventually lead to heart failure, arrhythmia, or heart attack.

4. Symptoms of coronary heart disease are chest pain, a pressing sensation on the chest, shortness of breath, pain in the arms or shoulder, lightheadedness, or pain in the jaw, neck, or back.

5. Metabolic Syndrome - This occurs when someone has a series of metabolic symptoms that put them at risk for coronary heart disease, stroke, or type 2 diabetes. When these symptoms occur together, it causes metabolic syndrome: abdominal obesity (belly fat), elevated triglycerides (blood fat disorders), high blood pressure, insulin resistance, glucose intolerance, increased risk to blood clotting, and the presence of an inflammatory state (there will be elevated C-reactive protein in the blood).

6. The main culprit in metabolic syndrome is excessive insulin in the body. This is caused by insulin resistance, which in turn creates an imbalance between glucose and insulin. The body's cells become resistant to insulin, bringing glucose into the cells, and the pancreas makes more and more insulin to try and

compensate.

7. Inflammation doesn't allow cells to absorb glucose, so it makes insulin resistance that much worse. Sugar levels rise and can get so high that they cause diabetes. Inflammation is the body's response to this insulin resistance, which creates increased levels of C-reactive protein. The next step is a higher risk of stroke and coronary heart disease.

Type 2 Diabetes

When your blood sugar is high, chemicals are released into your body that weakens your immune system, and inflammation takes the lead, trying to protect you. It often goes straight into overdrive, which raises the blood sugar even more, further weakening your immunity and perpetuating the cycle.

On a normal day, when you eat, your body breaks down carbs into glucose. That is a simple sugar that cruises in your blood and is used by tissues (such as muscle cells) as an energy source. Insulin is like the SWAT team that pulls in and regulates how much glucose stays behind in your blood. If too much glucose builds up, the pancreas releases more insulin.

Ideally, your pancreas produces just the right amount of insulin that your body needs. The body responds by taking in sugar and converting it to glucose, forming a well-functioning cycle.

Insulin resistance slows down the glucose access into your cells. Usually, inflammation is the culprit. It results in poor reception between the cells and the insulin signals, which causes more and more glucose to build up in the blood. This causes more inflammation, and the plot, quite literally, thickens.

Cancer

Inflammation can result in changes to our DNA. Researchers have found a link between these DNA shifts and colorectal cancer (Morris & Rossiter, 2011). Recurring infections (due to a decreased immune response) from viruses, bacteria, and yeast overgrowth can set the body up for developing growth and cancer cells. Certain strains of the human papilloma virus (HPV) increase the risk of cervical cancer.

Toxins in foods can stimulate cancer growth (which is why it is so important to eat more antioxidants).

If you already have growths or tumors, even if they are benign, inflammation can trigger them to grow larger, quicker. Processes that cause inflammation are the juice that makes all things swell and replicate - including cancer cells.

Cytokines are the cells that kick off inflammation. These are chemicals that send messages to cells to either enhance or suppress the immune system. The main responsibility of cytokines is to attack foreign cells or damaged tissue. This signals other parts of the immune system to get ready to go in with full force. Cytokines should naturally attack cancer cells, but the immune system doesn't recognize them as alien cells. So, they are left to grow out of control.

Asthma

Acute inflammation (the good type) is essential for the health of our lungs. We breathe in bacteria, viruses, and dust that float in the air around us. Inflammation naturally fights these tiny particles by producing an antibody called immunoglobulin E (IgE), and this breaks down the pollutants and toxins, keeping our lungs healthy.

People with asthma, however, have lungs and antibodies that overreact to irritants. Their immune systems produce way too many IgE antibodies, and these attach themselves to mast cells as part of their defense. When asthmatics inhale the irritant or particles, the antibodies latch on and force the mast cells to release histamine and leukotrienes in an attempt to eliminate the threat. These chemicals, however, irritate the lining of the lungs and airways. The airways constrict and spasm, which makes breathing much more difficult. The more the person tries to breathe, the more the airway is irritated, constricting it further.

These IgE reactions are one of the main causes of asthma. Another culprit is often sulfites, which are found in certain foods, dried fruit, and some wines.

Airway inflammation and asthma can be caused by allergic and non-allergic reactions.

Allergic asthma, also called extrinsic asthma, is triggered by allergens such as dog and cat hair, pet saliva, dust mites, mold, spores, and pollen.

Non-allergic asthma, or intrinsic asthma, is not an allergic reaction and can be triggered by multiple things - for example, smoke, paint fumes, smog, natural gas, and cooking fuel. It can also be brought on by exercises, respiratory infections, or changes in the weather.

Inflammatory Bowel Disease

Crohn's disease and ulcerative colitis are forms of inflammatory bowel disease that affect the colon and small intestine, inflaming sections of the gastrointestinal tract leading to serious complications.

Crohn's disease can occur anywhere in the gastrointestinal

tract and can even push into the bowel tissue layers. Sometimes, a healthy bowel is trapped between two inflamed, diseased areas.

Crohn's disease is believed to be an inflammatory reaction caused by building a protective layer around certain foods and falsely identifying some food types as 'invaders' and trying to eliminate them. The result is abdominal pain and diarrhea because the body is trying desperately to get rid of what it perceives as toxic.

Other symptoms of Crohn's disease include rectal bleeding (which can be so severe that it results in anemia), weight loss, fatigue, skin irritations, and fever. Surgery is required in two-thirds of Crohn's cases.

Ulcerative colitis forms ulcers and inflammation in the top lining of the colon and is quite common in the rectum. Symptoms are similar to Crohn's disease and can also include loss of appetite, bloody diarrhea mixed with mucus, skin lesions, and joint pain.

Inflammation can cause a number of other problems with the digestive tract, including leaky gut syndrome. This is when the protective layer between your gut and the outside world of your abdomen is compromised and microbes and other toxins' leak' out into your bloodstream. It can make you feel bloated and tired and, in severe cases, can be the cause of serious infection.

Autoimmune Disorders

When inflammation starts attacking your own cells, it can result in autoimmune disorders, which are basically diseases where your immune system sees normal body tissue as a threat. These disorders include lupus, rheumatoid arthritis, and multiple sclerosis. They appear to have a connection to the leaky gut syndrome, and people with autoimmune disorders also often have a deficiency in vitamin D. An anti-inflammatory diet can show remarkable improvement in these cases.

Lupus

Lupus can affect all organs but is primarily seen in the kidneys, skin, and joints. More than 90 percent of people who have lupus are women between the ages of 15 and 40, and it's largely determined by genetics.

Although lupus usually has a genetic predisposition, it can be triggered and worsened by diet, UV rays, penicillin, infections, exhaustion, stress, or a major injury. Lupus can be mild but can also be fatal, depending on the area of the body most affected.

- Brain and nervous system - symptoms may include headaches, personality changes, psychosis, tingling in the arms and legs, and seizures.

- Digestive tract - nausea, vomiting, and abdominal pain are most common here.

- Kidneys - signs to look out for include discolored urine and pain.

- Lungs - people with lupus may cough up blood.

- Skin - a common site for lupus symptoms and includes rashes (usually on the face).

General symptoms of lupus include fatigue, weight loss,

fever, mouth sores, and hair loss.

Although there is no cure for lupus, the symptoms can be kept under control with an anti-inflammatory diet.

Arthritis

The word 'arthritis' means inflammation of the joints. There are different types of arthritis, and most are the result of an immune response against the body (autoimmunity).

Common forms of arthritis that are due to an inflammatory response include rheumatoid arthritis, gout, systemic lupus erythematosus, and degenerative joint disease.

The symptoms are redness, swelling, joint pain, warm or hot areas, and limited ability to bend and move the joints.

Certain foods, like those in the nightshade family (potatoes, tomatoes, eggplant, and bell peppers), appear to contribute to inflammation in rheumatoid arthritis and osteoarthritis. This is usually due to an allergic response or heightened sensitivity to this family of vegetables.

Research shows that eating anti-inflammatory foods, such as fatty fish, results in a remarkable reduction in symptoms (Morris & Rossiter, 2011).

Osteoarthritis

In osteoarthritis, inflammation of the joints compresses the surrounding nerves, and the degeneration of the joint tissue diminishes the shock-absorbing ability of the area. It is an age-related form of arthritis. Osteoarthritis can be worsened with obesity or long-term overworking of a particular joint in work or sport.

Pain and other symptoms can be managed with medication, movement, adequate rest, proper hydration, and an anti-inflammatory diet.

Rheumatoid Arthritis

This autoimmune disease is caused by inflammation in the lining of smaller joints in the hands and feet. It can lead to bone deterioration and deformity. The disease often comes and goes, with periods of little to no pain and then sudden excruciating flare-ups.

Rheumatoid arthritis may be triggered by illness, bacteria and viruses, hormone imbalances, and smoking - all of which weaken the immune system.

It's important to follow an anti-inflammatory diet while being aware that some vegetables in the nightshade family may trigger symptoms to alleviate the symptoms. It's best to eliminate these to determine if it makes a difference. Interestingly, tobacco is also in the nightshade family, so if you're a smoker, that's the first thing you'll need to try to stop.

Multiple Sclerosis

In this debilitating illness, the body's immune system devours the protective covering around the nerves. This affects the communication between the brain and nerves and eventually leads to degeneration of the nerve tissue.

Early symptoms often include tingling in the arms and legs, fatigue, and dizziness. It progresses to vision problems (blurred, double, or loss) and strange 'shock' sensations when the head is moved in a certain way. In severe cases, people lose the ability to walk and talk.

Things that help soothe the symptoms include cooler weather (or a chilled bath), getting enough rest, exercise, and - you guessed it - an anti-inflammatory diet.

Now that you know how inflammation can affect your body, and after hearing a great deal about foods that can help alleviate some of the symptoms, it's time to take a closer look at diet.

4

FOODS THAT TRIGGER
INFLAMMATION

There are certain foods that not only trigger inflammation but can be a direct cause of a number of inflammatory diseases. It's fine to make an exception here and there, but for the most part, you'll want to avoid particular types of food.

In this chapter, we'll look at the 'bad' foods that cause inflammation, and we'll include a list of high-risk foods that should, ideally, be eliminated from your diet.

"Bad Foods" That Are Pro-Inflammation

Refined Sugars
Refined sugar is one of the leading culprits that trigger the

body's inflammatory response. It's not just in the spoons you stir into your coffee and sprinkle on your cereal. Sugar is also hidden in yogurt, salad dressings, and packaged foods. It can sneak in disguised as glucose or fructose and is difficult to eliminate because it is found in most foods that taste really good and give us a mood boost.

Several studies have connected the consumption of sugar, especially from sugary drinks, with chronic inflammation. People with diets high in refined sugar have more inflammatory markers, such as C-reactive protein, in their blood (Marengo, 2019). Researchers believe the inflammation is caused because sugar stimulates the production of free fatty acids in the liver and, when the body processes these acids, the resulting compounds can trigger inflammation.

In addition, when you eat sugar, it's broken down in your small intestines and released into your bloodstream. Insulin takes sugar from your blood and stores it in your cells. Insulin promotes the formation of arachidonic acid, which is a major component of pro-inflammatory cytokines (Gulbin, 2020). As sugar is acidic, the more you take in, the higher your system's pH will elevate. When your body is too acidic, it puts additional strain on your vital organs and triggers inflammation. This is also why you may feel your joints ache after eating too much-refined sugar.

Saturated Fats

Saturated fats are found in animal products such as red meat and full-fat dairy. These fats promote the release of endotoxin into the bloodstream, stimulating immune cells, which we now know leads directly to inflammation.

Your intestines contain more than 100 trillion microorganisms that assist with digestion. These little balls of life contain endotoxin in their cell walls. It's perfectly safe when they remain inside your gut and do their job, but they become problematic if they make their way into the bloodstream (Fritsche, 2015). Saturated fats promote the absorption of endotoxins from the intestines into the blood, instantly sounding alarm bells in your immune system.

Let's take a look at these individually.

Red Meat

There are compounds in red meat that increase its inflammatory profile dramatically. Eating red meat is associated with increased c-reactive protein (CRP), which is an inflammatory marker.

Trimethylamine oxide (TMAO) is produced in our bodies from carnitine, a substance found in animal muscle tissue. This chemical is linked to cardiovascular disease and inflammation. So, when we eat red meat, the bacteria in our gut break it down into molecules called trimethylamine (TMA), which is then processed in our liver, where it is converted to TMAO. Not only does it increase inflammation, but eating red meat on a regular basis also changes the microbiome in our gut.

Another tongue-twister associated with eating meat is advanced glycation end products (AGEs). They are formed when carbohydrates react with proteins and fats. When meats are browned on the grill, you can actually see this take place. It's called the Maillard reaction.

Higher levels of AGEs in our blood are directly linked to inflammation markers, including c-reactive protein and the homeostatic model assessment (HOMA) index, a known indicator of insulin resistance. High protein diets have higher amounts of AGEs. They are increased even more through processes like grilling and frying.

Research has also shown that AGEs are higher in women with polycystic ovary syndrome (PCOS), and this is linked with inflammation.

If you do eat red meat, you can lessen the impact by choosing high moisture cooking on lower heat and use acidic marinades that contain vinegar or lemon juice.

Dairy

There has been great controversy around whether dairy is a major contributor to chronic inflammation or not. It includes foods that are produced from the milk of cows and goats, such as cheese, butter, yogurt, ice cream, and kefir.

Before we look at inflammation, it's useful to take note of the benefits of dairy and how it contains some healthy nutrients (hence the controversy).

- It is packed with protein that is easily digested and absorbed. However, many people have lactose intolerance, making digestion problematic in these cases.

- Dairy is a rich source of calcium. We need calcium for nerve and muscle function and overall bone health.

- Cow's milk is often fortified with Vitamin D, which contributes to bone health, immune function, and, ironically, it also helps control inflammation.

- Yogurt and kefir are packed with probiotics that promote gut and immune health.

- Riboflavin (vitamin B2) and vitamin B12 are found in dairy, and these support energy, metabolism, and nerve function. Vegans typically need to take a vitamin B12 supplement because they eliminate meat and dairy from their diets.

- Dairy products are among the best sources of conjugated linoleic acid (CLA), which is a fatty acid connected to multiple health benefits.

But...

Dairy is also rich in saturated fats, which, as we discussed, are a leading trigger of inflammation. Dairy increases the absorption of inflammatory molecules called lipopolysaccharides, and research has shown that consuming dairy leads to increased acne, a common inflammatory condition (van der Walle, 2020).

Some of us also experience bloating, cramping, constipation, and diarrhea after eating dairy products. These symptoms also have a direct link to inflammation, although there are doctors who argue that it's more closely related to lactose intolerance.

There is research that supports both the inflammatory as well as anti-inflammatory effects of eating dairy. What appears to be in universal agreement is that individual dairy products have different impacts. For example, yogurt has been linked to a lower risk of type 2 diabetes (often associated with inflammation), and cheese consumption has been linked to a higher incidence of the same disease. Perhaps it's not dairy as a whole that needs to be avoided, but rather certain types.

It's also important to remember that every person's body is different, as is how we respond to specific foods. Dairy is one food group that you'll need to try out and test for yourself. Take note of your body's reactions after eating cheese one day and then perhaps after eating yogurt on a different day. Your individual body's wisdom is more important than general population research, especially when it's contradictory.

However, it is worthy to note that the benefits you may gain from eating dairy are also available from other food groups, and your body won't suffer any harm from eliminating it.

Starches and Carbohydrates

A massive part of reducing inflammation comes down to understanding your starches. An anti-inflammatory diet isn't just about eating more fish and greens. The grains you take in can have an even bigger impact.

Carbohydrates are an important source of energy and the only source of dietary fiber. Fiber reduces inflammation and improves your gut health. Whole grains also contain powerful antioxidants and bioactive compounds that help to reduce free radical damage and inflammation.

However, some carbs have the opposite effect. Refined starches that are low in fiber can spike your blood sugar, and some starchy treats, like cupcakes, have additional sugar that also kicks your inflammation up a few notches. Eating too many processed starches can also lead to weight gain, which is directly linked to inflammatory responses.

Carbohydrates are like the throttle behind inflammation. They can keep blood sugar slow and steady, decreasing inflammation, or they can rev a sudden spike that shoots inflammation right up again.

Here are the carbs you want to avoid:

- Donuts and pastries - In addition to the refined flour, these are laden with full-fat butter and sweet glazing - a definite no-go zone.

- Muffins and bagels - They sound healthy but usually contain refined flour.

- Simple starches such as white potatoes, white rice, white pasta, and white bread.

- Cereals with added sugar or corn syrup

- Anything made with refined flour: pretzels, pancakes, biscuits, tortillas, waffles, cakes, and so on.

Omega-6 Fatty Acids

Omega-6 fatty acids are good for you. They are mainly found in vegetable oils and help lower harmful LDL cholesterol and boost the good, protective high-density lipoprotein (HDL) cholesterol. They also improve the body's response to insulin, helping to keep your blood sugar balanced.

However, they need to be eaten in the correct ratio to omega-3 fatty acids. If the scale is tipped and you're taking in a lot of omega-6 but not enough omega-3 to balance it out, the results can be increased inflammation.

The main problem with omega-6 fatty acids is that the body converts linolenic acid (the most common omega-6) into arachidonic acid. This is the building block for molecules that promote inflammation which we actually need (it helps blood clotting after injury, for instance). But, in excess, it can lead to constriction of the blood vessels.

On average, Americans eat 10 times more omega-6 fats than omega-3s- that's the problem; not the fact that they have healthy omega-6 in their bodies. Improve the ratio of omega-3 to omega-6, and you're good to go. Eat more threes - don't eat fewer sixes.

Artificial Sweeteners

Synthetic sugar substitutes are the real villains when it comes to inflammation. Ironically, we often opt for diet sodas, sweeteners in our coffee, and low-calorie sweets because we are trying to lose weight and be 'healthy.' Sadly, artificial sweeteners come at a high cost to the rest of our health.

Sweeteners are processed by our liver and create a toxic effect in our body, sending a message to our brains that we are still hungry. This spikes our insulin, and we tend to eat more.

In addition to tampering with our hunger levels, artificial sweeteners are known, inflammatory-inducing culprits. It's best to avoid them altogether. Try natural alternatives such as honey or brown rice syrup instead.

The Hidden Danger of Preservatives

Additives and preservatives are added to processed foods to thicken or stabilize them. It helps food producers keep products on the shelf longer and helps us when we cook because some emulsifiers thicken sauces. Emulsifiers also help ice cream stay creamy.

However, many of these additives disrupt the bacteria in the gastrointestinal tract and lead to inflammation. Boxes or cans of food that contain more than five ingredients on the label are usually the culprits.

Avoid highly processed foods and opt for fresh products that are in their natural, raw state. Artificially flavored, highly preserved foods should ideally be eliminated.

In a nutshell, you'll want to steer clear of the following: loaves of bread, waffles, pancakes, bagels, baked goods, cereals (except for oatmeal), corn syrup, tortillas, sodas, fried foods, hard cheeses, ice cream, and frozen yogurt, jams and jellies, pasta, potatoes, processed meat, red meat, and sugary treats.

Usually, the less 'natural' a food is, and the more ingredients it contains, the more inflammatory it is. Look at the labels of the food you buy and be aware of words such as refined, enriched, or processed.

Fortunately, there are plenty of healthy alternatives. Some foods are not only "not inflammatory," they actually decrease inflammation as well. We'll take a look at these in the next chapter.

5

ANTI-INFLAMMATORY FOODS

Many delicious foods can help you fight inflammation. They are perfect for your gut health, will help reduce your aches and pains, and you'll likely feel far less tired in just a few days.

In this chapter, we'll look at the 'good' foods that decrease inflammation. We'll include a list of foods that you can start including in your diet that will make an immediate positive difference.

"Good Foods" That Decrease Inflammation

Omega 3 Fatty Acids

Long-chain omega-3 fatty acids, known as eicosapentaenoic

acid (EPA) and docosahexaenoic acid (DHA), are metabolized by the body into compounds called resolvins and protectins. These are known to reduce inflammation.

Rich sources of these omega-3 fatty acids include the following fatty fish:

- salmon

- sardines

- herring

- mackerel

- anchovies

You can also find omega-3 in the following non-fishy alternatives:

- chia seeds

- hemp

- flaxseeds and flaxseed oil

- pumpkin seeds

- walnuts

Broccoli Sprouts

Eating large amounts of broccoli, cauliflower, Brussels sprouts, and kale (cruciferous vegetables) has been proven to decrease heart disease and cancer risk. The antioxidants they contain are responsible for anti-inflammatory effects. Broccoli, in particular, is one of the best sources of sulforaphane, an antioxidant that reduces your body's levels of cytokines and (here comes a mouthful) nuclear factor kappa-light-chain-enhancer (NF-kB), known drivers of inflammation.

Carrots

Orange veggies are known to be rich in Vitamin A and beta-carotene, which fight inflammation. Interestingly, cooking appears to increase the absorption of these compounds. Add carrots, squash, and sweet potatoes to your dinner plate regularly.

Green Leafy Vegetables

Leafy greens have substantial concentrations of vitamins and nutrients that are known to reduce chronic inflammation. Vitamin A, D, E, and K, and alpha-linolenic acid, are present in the healthy, almost calorie-free leaves.

These veggies include spinach, kale, chard, arugula, turnip greens, beet greens, Brussels sprouts, asparagus, and collard greens.

Here are some anti-inflammatory tips:

- The darker the greens, the better. This is usually indicative of higher nutrient content. For example, opt for baby spinach leaves instead of iceberg lettuce.

- Be generous with extra virgin olive oil when eating them. Many of the vitamins can only be absorbed when paired with oil. This simple dressing (perhaps combined with balsamic vinegar) is a much better choice than fat-free salad dressing.

- Try to eat most of the greens raw. It may feel easier to digest when the leaves are cooked, but this comes at the cost of losing very important nutrients. Olive oil also breaks down at high temperatures and loses its beneficial qualities.

You don't have to simply stick to salads, however. Sneak some leaves on a whole-grain sandwich, add them to a healthy green smoothie, toss liberally on scrambled eggs, or roast with other types of vegetables (include onions and garlic for an extra anti-inflammatory boost).

Other Vegetables

While most vegetables are nutritional and exceptionally good for your health overall, these ones stand out as the best inflammation fighters:

- Sweet potatoes and squash. These contain carotenoids like beta-cryptoxanthin and are rich in antioxidants. Beta-cryptoxanthin may reduce your risk of developing rheumatoid arthritis and other inflammatory conditions.

- Red and green peppers. Whether they're mild or hot, green, yellow or red, they're abundant in vitamin C. This helps strengthen bones and can protect cartilage (great for arthritis).

- Squash

Citrus Fruits

Citrus fruits are packed with vitamin C, and this is vital for the synthesis of collagen. Collagen helps to build and repair blood vessels, tendons, ligaments, and even bone. For this reason, it offers relief for different types of arthritis. Citrus fruits are also excellent sources of antioxidants that fight many other inflammatory conditions.

The types of citrus fruits you can include in your diet are oranges, grapefruit, lemon, and lime. You can have this in juice form, eaten as whole fruit along with your breakfast, or simply by squeezing some lime or lemon juice over your food (it's perfect with salmon).

Pineapple

Pineapples are rich in vitamin C and bromelain, which is an enzyme that has been linked to decreased pain and swelling in osteoarthritis and rheumatoid arthritis. Bromelain is an anti-inflammatory gem and is perfect in this form.

When it's pushed in higher quantities, as a supplement, for example, it can have other detrimental effects if you're taking blood-thinners for other conditions. Bromelain in these higher doses can increase the risk of bleeding and may also affect the efficacy of antibiotics and sedatives.

Eating pineapple, however, is harmless and gives you just the right amount. Toss some cubes in a fruit salad, add pieces to sweet and sour dishes, blend into a smoothie, or slice some into a healthy stir-fry.

Fiber

Your body needs soluble and insoluble fiber.

Soluble fiber binds with water to form a gel which slows down digestion. This helps your body absorb nutrients and plays a role in lowering cholesterol, particularly bad (LDL) cholesterol. Soluble fiber is found in foods such as nuts, seeds, beans, lentils, oat bran, and barley.

Insoluble fiber adds bulk to your stool, makes you feel fuller, and helps food move through your digestive tract. It also aids in preventing constipation. Excellent sources of insoluble fiber include vegetables, whole grains, legumes, and wheat bran.

It's been shown that if you have a diet that is high in fiber, you'll have lower levels of C-reactive protein in your blood (that useful marker for inflammation). It also helps reduce inflammation by helping to keep body weight down, and high-fiber foods feed beneficial bacteria in your colon. They, in turn, release substances that lower levels of inflammation all around your body.

Prebiotics are a type of fiber found in certain plants that are excellent at reducing inflammation. These are the types of foods to include: onions, garlic, oats, banana, artichokes, and dandelion root.

Overall, you need between 20 and 30 grams of fiber per day (soluble and insoluble). Aim to fill at least a quarter of your plate at each meal with whole grains. Here are some fantastic options that include the entire grain kernel: bulgur, oatmeal, whole cornmeal, and brown rice. Half of your plate needs to be filled with fruits or vegetables, which leaves just a quarter for protein.

Always drink plenty of water because this helps the fiber work more effectively.

If you're sensitive to gluten, found in wheat and other grains, certain fibers may trigger inflammation in your body. It may be worth testing for celiac disease or a wheat allergy and sticking to other fiber options such as oats and rice.

Herbal Teas

- Green tea is rich in catechins that have strong anti-inflammatory effects. It's high in antioxidants that assist in reducing free radicals and combat oxidative stress (which is an accelerator of the aging process). In addition to decreasing inflammation, green tea has other benefits, such as fighting harmful bacteria and viruses.

- Rooibos tea, also called red bush tea, is naturally sweet and caffeine-free. It contains flavonoids, an antioxidant that reduces symptoms of inflammation.

- Turmeric tea is a vibrant orange-gold. Turmeric contains curcumin which reduces inflammation.

Fermented Foods

Around 80 percent of your body's immune tissue is in your digestive tract. The bacteria in your gut is one of the most important influencers of healthy digestion. Probiotics - which is food to your microbiome - increase your energy levels, reduce inflammation, and support your immune system.

Fermented foods are powerful natural sources of probiotics. In addition, the acidic by-products of fermentation promote the breakdown of macro and micronutrients in your diet, which helps to reduce bloating and stomach cramps. Many vegetables are even more nutritious after fermenting than they are when they're raw or cooked.

One important thing to note before we go on, however, is that if you haven't already been including fermented foods in your diet, start off slowly. They are incredibly strong and can cause uncomfortable reactions in your bowel if you eat too much all at once.

Here are some fermented food options worth trying:

- Kombucha is made from a symbiotic colony of bacteria and yeast (SCOBY) and mixed with sweetened black or green tea. While fermenting, the SCOBY digests sugars in the tea and produces B vitamins and probiotic bacteria. SCOBY contains Saccharomyces boulardii, which has a positive effect on digestion and skin conditions such as dermatitis. Polyphenol compounds from tea can help reduce cholesterol levels, decrease blood sugar, and even reduce the risk of certain cancers.

- Kimchi is a Korean favorite and a leading source of probiotics. It's made by fermenting cabbage with probiotic lactic acid bacteria. Use it on top of sandwiches or as a barbecue side. It not only decreases inflammation but is also known to reduce the risk of metabolic syndrome and certain cancers.

- Kefir is much like yogurt but thinner and tangier. It's made from fermenting milk using kefir grains. It's rich in the beneficial bacteria, Lactobacillus higarii. It's way more beneficial than standard yogurt and has more probiotics that promote healthy digestion and a very happy microbiome. It also contains B vitamins and tryptophan, an amino acid that is a building block for the mood-stabilizing hormone serotonin. Add some flavor and sweetness with cinnamon and berries.

- Pickled fruit and vegetables. The pickling process preserves food in salty water (brine) or vinegar. Choose pickles that are also lacto-fermented, and you'll want them to be raw and unpasteurized. Pickled onions are a really good bet!

- Sauerkraut. This is a great source of fiber, has immune-boosting vitamin C and bone-building vitamin K. It should be raw and unpasteurized (you'll find it in the refrigerator) and not canned. Pasteurization kills beneficial bacteria. Even better than hunting through jars in the shops, why not make it yourself? We've included a handy and easy recipe in this book.

- Miso is wildly popular in Asia for its savory, umami flavor. It's a rich source of iron, calcium, potassium, B vitamins, and protein. It contains a strain of bacteria that has been linked to reducing symptoms of inflammatory bowel disease. Be careful to add it at the end of the cooking process (for example, in miso soup) because heat kills all that good bacteria.

- Tempeh is made from fermented soybeans. It's a complete protein and a brilliant addition to any vegan's diet. It takes on the flavor of anything it is cooked with, making it truly versatile in the kitchen. Tempeh supports muscle growth and repair, improves bone strength, and reduces inflammation and cholesterol levels. Soy foods are also rich in omega-3 fatty acids, so it's a win-win.

Ginger

Ginger not only reduces inflammation, but it's a powerhouse for fighting other chronic conditions too. A 2014 study found that volatile ginger oil reduced the symptoms of ulcerative colitis, which is an inflammatory bowel disease (Laboratories, n.d.).

It's also been shown to decrease renal inflammation and offers relief for people with chronic kidney disease. It improves diet-induced metabolic abnormalities and can slow down the growth of some cancers (including breast cancer).

It's a fantastic home remedy for women suffering from regular urinary tract infections (UTIs) as well. It alkalizes your urine, making it less acidic. This dramatically reduces the burning sensation experienced with a UTI.

Use fresh ginger in your dressings, teas, juices, smoothies, and dishes. It's a powerful herb, and you may even notice a shift in your digestive response the first time you use it.

If you have particularly slow digestion, use a pinch of freshly grated ginger with every meal. You can gradually increase this to over a teaspoon each time. You can do this every day for the rest of your life, and there are usually no adverse effects - only good results. You only need to be cautious if you are on medications to help blood clotting, as ginger does affect blood flow in larger doses.

Ginger keeps your gut healthy and also lends a hand in stabilizing blood sugar, eases nausea and motion sickness, decreases flatulence, and works wonders for those debilitating 24-hour stomach bugs.

Curcumin

This substance, found in the ginger family, is the force behind turmeric, often used in curries. It is a powerful anti-inflammatory and has shown to be of particular benefit for patients with rheumatoid and osteoarthritis. Research has shown that curcumin is just as effective as ibuprofen at reducing joint pain and swelling in some cases (Laboratories, n.d.).

Although you can certainly add turmeric to curries for the anti-inflammatory benefit, it's also easily added for some orange-colored zing to juices and smoothies.

Onions

Similar to garlic, onions have a high sulfur content. They are antiviral and antibacterial and have a particularly positive effect on symptoms associated with atherosclerosis (hardened arteries). Onions are also packed with fructooligosaccharides which positively influence gut health. Try and chop a few into at least one meal a day.

Mushrooms

Mushrooms are not only anti-inflammatory, but they are also rich in protein, vitamins, minerals, antioxidants, and amino acids. They also contain polysaccharides that are excellent for your immune system. The best ones to pick off the shelf include Asian, maitake, oyster, and shiitake mushrooms. These should be cooked and not eaten raw. They contain no fats, are filling, and also help decrease cholesterol.

Mushrooms also contain linoleic acid, which has an anti-carcinogenic effect and helps fight certain cancers. In addition, they're loaded with calcium, vitamin D, iron, potassium, and selenium. These lower your blood pressure, fight anemia and strengthen your bones.

To summarize, you'll want to include more of the following foods in your diet: fruit and vegetables (excluding the nightshade family), fatty fish, green leafy veggies, key spices, mushrooms, onions, fermented foods, and good old fiber.

If this is very different from how you usually eat, you may be concerned about how you are going to prepare your meals and incorporate these new food choices. In the next chapter, we'll dive into different ways to include anti-inflammatory ingredients easily, how to make smart choices when dining out, and how to combine your foods for the best effect.

6

THE ANTI-INFLAMMATORY DIET

Changing your diet may feel daunting, especially if you've been used to a completely different way of eating. But this is your chance for a new beginning and a healthier lifestyle. You'll feel better, live longer, and enjoy your meals more, knowing that they are nutritious and good for you.

Instead of thinking of the anti-inflammatory diet as being restrictive, see it as an opportunity and a challenge. Start slowly - even adding just a few healthy ingredients each day and eliminating one bad choice every other week will make a huge difference.

In this chapter, we'll look at when and how to eat for maximum benefit, easy ways to incorporate anti-inflammatory foods, and how to make smart choices when dining out and traveling.

Know Your Cooking Oils

You want to try and avoid cooking in high-fat butter. There is a range of healthier choices. We'll have a brief look here:

Olive Oil

This monounsaturated fat contains iron, vitamin K, and antioxidants (which help lower the risk of cancer and heart disease). Extra-virgin olive oil decreases inflammation, is antibacterial, assists with insulin resistance, and helps to retain the anti-inflammatory properties of the other foods you are cooking.

Note that non-virgin olive oils don't have the same antioxidant benefits.

Avocado Oil

You'll notice the recipes later in the book often include avocado oil - and for a good reason. Avocado oil is rich in oleic acid, reduces cholesterol, neutralizes free radicals, improves heart health, is high in lutein (brilliant for your eyes), enhances the absorption of nutrients in other foods, reduces arthritic symptoms, improves skin, and even speeds up the healing of wounds.

Sesame Oil

Sesame oil is rich in essential fatty acids and helps to lower cholesterol. It has a high linoleic acid content, which helps prevent inflammatory conditions such as arthritis, hair loss, mood swings, and even heart disease. Go for the unrefined sesame oils, as these are also packed with antioxidants. This oil is high in omega-6 fatty acids, so you'll need to balance out with omega-3s in your diet.

Sunflower Oil

Sunflower oil is the one that is highest in vitamin E. Vitamin E is known to reduce the risk of cancer and heart disease. Look for high oleic sunflower oil, and remember, just like sesame oil, it's high in omega-6, so it needs to be balanced out with extra omega-3s.

Coconut Oil

Even though coconut oil is 90 percent saturated fat (which would usually be a bad thing), half of that fat is lauric acid. This is known to prevent heart disease, and the oil is also anti-aging, great for your hair and skin, and is also a powerful antioxidant. It makes a great substitute for butter in recipes.

When and How to Eat

Intermittent Fasting

Our bodies respond well to periods of not eating or eating less (smaller portions). Intermittent fasting (IF) or time-restricted feeding (TRF) has shown positive results for people struggling with chronic inflammation. Both IF and TRF enhances autophagy, which is your body's ability to clean out dead and dysfunctional cells. This, in turn, lowers inflammation. When your body gets a break from digesting food, it has a chance to eliminate waste and dedicate its focus to cleansing.

It doesn't mean you need to starve yourself. Simply stop eating after a certain time (for example, 6 pm) and only start eating a minimum of 12 hours later (in this case, the next morning at 6 am). If you're able to narrow that window, even more, all the better.

This does mean no more midnight snacks, but your

digestion will feel better almost instantly, and you'll probably notice your inflammation symptoms cooling down too.

Easy Ways to Incorporate Anti-Inflammatory Foods in Your Diet

You don't need to radically change your diet overnight. You can slowly start bringing in foods that have an anti-inflammatory effect and decrease the pro-inflammatory foods bit by bit. It doesn't have to involve bizarre new recipes or a whole new way of eating. There are some simple things you can do that will have a massive effect:

Spice Things Up

Add fragrant and pungent spices to your meals, such as a little garlic, to your dinner this evening. Herbs and spices such as turmeric, rosemary, cinnamon, cumin, ginger, and fenugreek decrease inflammation and can easily be added to most dishes. You'll probably enjoy your meals so much more, too, because they add a dash of flavor and warmth.

Garlic is one of the best anti-inflammatory secrets. It contains quercetin, a chemical that naturally inhibits histamine (a known trigger for inflammation), and also contains sulfur compounds that strengthen your immune system. Garlic provides almost instant relief for arthritic pain and swelling.

Ginger contains gingerols, a substance that reduces inflammation and tones down pain in the body. It also supports digestion and peristalsis, has been proven to reduce colorectal cancer, and keeps the microbes in your gut happy.

Think Mediterranean

A Mediterranean-style diet is considered the top anti-inflammatory way of eating. It consists mainly of fresh fruit and vegetables, nuts, seeds, and seafood. These are packed not only with essential nutrients and minerals but also antioxidants and omega-3 fatty acids that help reduce inflammation.

Try to go for gluten-free options when it comes to the sides of bread that are often included in the recipes, as gluten can trigger inflammation if you have an intolerance or sensitivity to it.

Berries on Your Breakfast

Berries contain antioxidants known as anthocyanins. This is what gives them their bright red, blue, and purple colors. Anthocyanins are brilliant at fighting inflammation, and they also train our cells to respond faster to future inflammatory episodes.

It's easy to start adding berries to your diet. Simply sprinkle a few on your oats in the morning. You can enjoy the sweetness of blueberries, raspberries, blackberries, or strawberries and get tremendous anti-inflammatory effects at the same time.

Add Some Green to Every Meal

Each time you prepare a meal, try to make at least half of it green. Keep these leafy greens in your refrigerator or herb garden: spinach, kale, Swiss chard, arugula, and dandelion greens. These are almost calorie-free, filled with vitamins and fiber, are rich in antioxidants, and have an alkalizing effect on the body - brilliant for decreasing inflammation.

Something Fishy

If you're used to eating lots of red meat, try replacing one of these servings each week with a piece of fish instead. Salmon and other fatty fish are high in omega-3 and have significant anti-inflammatory effects that are noticed almost instantly. This is a particularly important substitute for red meat if you have an autoimmune condition such as lupus, rheumatoid arthritis, or multiple sclerosis.

An Avo a Day

Avocados are laden with monounsaturated, 'good,' fats which reduce cholesterol and calm inflammation. They are also high in vitamin K, C, and E, and zinc. Zinc is an antioxidant and anti-inflammatory, and studies have shown that zinc supplements decreased infections, oxidative stress, and inflammatory cytokines in the elderly (Prasad, 2014). Avocados have also been shown to be beneficial in preventing neurodegenerative diseases such as Alzheimer's and Parkinson's. So, slice one up each day and add it to a whole grain sandwich, chop it into your salad, or blend one into your smoothie.

Chow Some Chia

Chia seeds are called a superfood for a reason. They are one of the best sources of fiber in the world, and fiber is essential for balancing blood sugar and keeping your gut healthy. They are also loaded with antioxidants and omega-3 fatty acids. Just a spoonful in your smoothie added to a quinoa dish, or sprinkled on your oats, makes this an easy addition to any diet.

Dining Out and Traveling

Cooking at home is one thing, but what happens when you're in a different country or eating out at a restaurant?

Menus often include hidden inflammatory foods, and making healthy choices can seem overwhelming and complicated. It becomes even more challenging when eating out with friends and seeing all the tempting food on their plates.

It helps to view the menu beforehand, if possible so that you're prepared. Most restaurants have these available on their websites. Planning is the main part of your success.

Here are some tips to help you navigate the menu.

Skip the Bread

Breadsticks, rolls, and other bonus carbs for the table are tempting but an unnecessary inflammatory injection. Rather, skip the bread and order a shared salad for the table.

Dressing on the Side

When ordering your meals and salads, opt to have your dressings and sauces on the side (or skip them altogether). These are usually rich in cream and saturated fat. Having it on the side allows you to have a small taste while leaving most of it untouched. Choose extra-virgin olive oil and balsamic vinegar for your salads instead of the rich alternatives.

Salad not Fries

Most restaurants allow you to select your side (when ordering meat, for example). Instead of going for potatoes or fries, choose veggies or a salad. Also, remember that not all salads are equal. Try to go for a standard green salad. The dense, fancy salads that include croutons, rich dressing, egg, and pasta are full of inflammatory gremlins.

Fish, Fish, Fish

Grilled fish will always be a better decision than red meat

or fried chicken. Steer away from the fatty beer batter and be liberal with the lemon and lime juice. Try to choose fatty fish as much as possible. Salmon is your ideal choice.

Opt for Variety

Some restaurants have very large portion sizes with limited variety on the plate. It's often smarter to order two or three starters instead of one main. That allows you to have a selection of healthy bite-sized options, almost like an anti-inflammatory buffet. Starters are also often healthier and lower in calories. For example, order a green salad, grilled chicken strips, and some mushrooms.

Be Wise with Your Drinks

Try to stick to sparkling water instead of sodas or fruit juice. When it comes to alcohol, wine is a healthier alternative to beers, ciders, and mixes.

Delectable Desserts - No Need to Skip Them

You don't need to go without dessert, but try to go for healthier options such as fruit salad, sorbet, or a special type of coffee. Always opt for 'lighter' - for example, a fluffy dark chocolate mousse is usually a better choice than a dense piece of chocolate cake.

Restaurant Menu Tricks

- Avoid any menu items that include the following words: cured, battered, breaded, batter-dipped, or tempura.

- Say yes to terms such as baked, poached, boiled, grilled, and steamed.

- Find out if the restaurant will allow adult ordering of a kid's dish - this is usually more appropriate in terms of portion size.

Restriction Versus Elimination

This isn't a diet, and it's not a punishment. You're not eliminating certain foods to get to a number on a scale. You're eliminating chronic inflammation so that you can live a happier, healthier life. You're giving yourself the greatest gift. Imagine waking up pain-free, without feeling sluggish in the morning. Think about eliminating brain fog as opposed to eliminating that piece of cake.

Also, remember that this entire process is trial and error according to how your body responds. Some foods may have to be removed from your diet forever (especially if you have an allergy, intolerance, or sensitivity). Some foods might only be removed for a short period of time as your body learns to find its balance again (you may be able to reintroduce certain foods you used to have a reaction to - such as a particular type of vegetable or cooking oil).

Elimination should be thought of as substitution. You're not just excluding red meat from your diet. For instance, you're introducing grilled fish. It's a good trade, not a sacrifice.

Some foods don't have to be eliminated completely but rather restricted. Consider eating red meat only once a week, for example, as opposed to every night. Perhaps you treat yourself to a sweet treat on a Sunday, but the rest of the week, you avoid refined sugars. Ultimately, it's about finding balance

- in your mind, your body, and your lifestyle.

Let's fixate on all the delicious, healing foods that you CAN eat. The next chapter provides you with 10 anti-inflammatory recipes that will make you forget you're cutting out anything at all.

7

10 WHOLESOME ANTI-INFLAMMATORY RECIPES

Now that you know what types of foods you should cut down on, as well as which foods you need to start adding for the ultimate anti-inflammatory benefits, you may be wondering what this looks like on your plate every day. We've included 10 anti-inflammatory recipes in this chapter. There are some side dishes or snacks, a couple of examples for breakfast, lunch, and dinner, and even some dessert! They're simple to make, taste delicious, and pack a hefty anti-inflammatory punch.

Let's dig in!

Gingerbread with Gumption Oatmeal

Oatmeal is rich in antioxidants, high in fiber, lowers cholesterol, and helps reduce blood pressure. It also provides half the requirements of your daily omega-3s, and ginger is an excellent anti-inflammatory.

Ingredients

- 4 cups of water

- 2 cups of old-fashioned oats (don't use the quick-cooking type)

- 1 ½ tablespoon ground cinnamon

- ¼ teaspoon ground coriander

- ¼ teaspoon ground cloves

- ¼ teaspoon ground ginger

- ¼ teaspoon ground allspice

- ¼ teaspoon ground cardamom

- ⅛ teaspoon ground nutmeg

- Sweetener or honey according to taste

- Berries of your choice to sprinkle on top

Method

1. Bring water to the boil in a pot.

2. Add the oats and spices.

3. Stir occasionally until the oats are done.

4. Serve with honey and berries.

You can freeze any leftover oats in muffin tins and, once frozen, keep them in freezer-safe zipper-top bags. This gives you single servings that you can pop out and reheat.

Tasty Turmeric Scrambled Eggs with Spinach

This is a simple and healthy breakfast that is easy to whip up. You should try and limit your egg breakfasts to a maximum of two a week, however. Eggs are best in moderation.

Ingredients
- 3 large eggs

- 2 cups raw baby spinach leaves

- 1 tablespoon coconut oil

- 1 teaspoon turmeric

- Salt and pepper to taste

Method
1. Whisk the eggs and turmeric together in a bowl.

2. Melt the coconut oil in a non-stick frying pan.

3. Add the spinach and mix through the oil until it has wilted.

4. Add the turmeric eggs mixture and combine with the spinach.

5. Using a spatula or wooden spoon, move the eggs to the center of the pan. Do this continuously until they are cooked. It usually only takes two to three minutes.

6. Remove from the heat and season with salt and pepper.

7. For some added anti-inflammatory benefits, add mushrooms, avocado, baby tomato, or salmon to your plate.

8. Serve with rosemary sprigs and a side of orange juice.

Smoked Salmon Salad with Magic Green Dressing

Salmon is one of the best sources of omega-3 fatty acids, and this recipe is gluten-free and low in calories.

Ingredients

- ½ cup of green lentils

- 2 thinly sliced baby fennel bulbs (save some leaves too)

- ½ cup natural yogurt

- 2 tablespoons chopped parsley

- 2 tablespoons chopped chives

- 1 tablespoon chopped tarragon

- 1 tablespoon salted baby capers (rinsed and drained)

- 1 teaspoon finely grated lemon rind

- ½ thinly sliced red onion

- 1 tablespoon lemon juice

- Pinch of castor sugar

- ½ avocado (sliced)

- 2 ounces baby spinach (about a handful)

- 7 ounces smoked salmon (sliced)

Method

1. Cook the lentils in boiling water for 20 minutes or until tender. Drain and keep aside.

2. While the lentils are cooking, heat a pan over high heat—Cook fennel slices in a thin layer of olive oil for about two minutes on each side.

3. Blend the yogurt, parsley, chives, tarragon, capers, and lemon rind in a food processor until smooth. Add pepper to taste. This is your magic green dressing!

4. Place onion, juice, sugar, and salt in a bowl. Set aside for five minutes and then drain.

5. Combine the lentils, fennel, onion, spinach, and avocado in a bowl. Top with salmon and sprinkle with fennel leaves and parsley. Drizzle with the magic green dressing.

6. Serve and enjoy!

Black Bean Buddha Bowl With Creamy Cashew Dressing

Black beans are high in protein, fill you up, and are surprisingly low in calories. That is also why we can afford to add this decadent and very yummy dressing! This anti-inflammatory bowl will have you coming back for seconds.

Ingredients

- 1 cup of quinoa (rinsed and drained)

- 2 ⅓ cups of water

- 2 tablespoons ground cumin

- 2 tablespoons extra virgin olive oil

- 1 red onion (finely chopped)

- 2 crushed garlic cloves

- 2 teaspoons sweet paprika

- 400g can of black beans (rinsed and drained)

- 2 zucchinis (cut into thin strips)

- Kernels from 2 corn cobs

- 1 thinly sliced red chili

- Fresh coriander leaves for serving

Coriander and Cashew Dressing Ingredients

- 2 ounces of raw cashews (soak in cold water for three hours)

- 1 tablespoon lemon juice

- 1 tablespoon extra-virgin olive oil

- 2 tablespoons chopped coriander

- ¼ cup of water

Method

1. Boil the quinoa, 2 cups of water, and 1 tablespoon of cumin. Once boiling, reduce heat to low and cook for 12 minutes, or until the quinoa is al dente.

2. Heat oil in a saucepan over medium heat. Add the onion and cook until it has softened. Now add the garlic, paprika, and remaining cumin—Cook and stir for one minute. Add the black beans and remaining water and simmer until all the water has evaporated. Mash the beans into coarse pieces with a fork.

3. To prepare the dressing, drain the cashews, which you soaked for three hours. Blend the cashews, lemon juice, oil, and coriander in a food processor. Gradually add water until it is thick and creamy.

4. Divide the quinoa, beans, zucchini, and corn among the bowls to serve. Drizzle with the creamy cashew dressing, and sprinkle with chili and coriander.

Easy Roasted Tomato Chicken Breasts

Tomatoes are rich in lycopene and vitamin C and are one of the top defeaters of inflammation. You may need to be careful if you suffer from any form of arthritis, however. Check your sensitivity to nightshade veggies, as tomatoes may flare up your inflammation if you are prone to reactions with this food group.

Ingredients

- 2 chicken breasts (with skin)

- 1 teaspoon black pepper

- 2 tablespoons extra virgin olive oil

- salt to taste

- 32 ounces cherry tomatoes

- 2 (15 ounces) cans of cannellini beans (drained and rinsed)

- 1 cup pitted olives

- 1 teaspoon lemon zest from one lemon

- 1 teaspoon chopped rosemary leaves

Method

1. Preheat the oven to 425 degrees Fahrenheit.

2. Cut chicken breasts in half and crosswise.

3. Season chicken pieces with pepper and salt then set aside.

4. Stir olive oil, tomatoes, beans, olives, lemon zest, and rosemary together in a baking dish.

5. Place seasoned chicken breast pieces (skin side up) on top of tomato mixture.

6. Bake in the preheated oven until chicken is cooked through, stirring vegetables about halfway through. It usually takes around 50 minutes.

7. Serve with a side of roasted vegetables (with plenty of garlic and onions).

Ground Turkey Bowl with Mushroom Cabbage Rice

This is a low-carb, filling, and wholesome recipe that is filled with anti-inflammatory ingredients. Turkey is also a wonderful alternative to red meat. You don't have to only eat fish and chicken!

Turkey Ingredients

- 2 tablespoons avocado oil

- 1 small diced onion

- 1 apple (peeled and cored)

- 5 cloves garlic, minced

- 2 cups chopped mushrooms

- 1 pound ground turkey

- 2 zucchini squash (chopped)

- 2 teaspoons dried or fresh oregano

- 1 teaspoon ground ginger

- 1 teaspoon salt

- 4 cups baby spinach leaves

Cabbage Rice Ingredients

- 2 tablespoons avocado oil

- 1 large head of grated green cabbage

- ½ teaspoon sea salt, to taste

Method

Cabbage Rice Preparation:

1. Chop the cabbage into chunks and pulse in a food processor until the pieces are rice-sized.

2. Heat the avocado oil in a large skillet or wok. Add the cabbage rice, cover with a lid, and cook on medium heat while stirring frequently. The cabbage will soften and turn golden brown in about eight minutes.

Turkey Preparation:

1. Heat the avocado oil over medium-high heat and add the onion and apple.

2. Cook until the onion turns translucent.

3. Add the mushrooms and cook for a further three minutes.

4. Keep the vegetables aside.

5. Brown the ground turkey, and then add the vegetables.

6. Add the remaining ingredients and stir well.

7. Cover and cook for five minutes, or until the turkey is cooked through and the zucchini is soft. Add salt to taste.

8. Serve with cabbage rice.

9. You can also add other veggies such as broccoli, cauliflower, Brussels sprouts, kale, and sweet potato.

10. If you're not a turkey fan, replace it with ground chicken or a vegan mince alternative.

Tantalizing Turmeric Chicken Soup

Few things are as comforting as warm, spicy chicken soup, especially if you're feeling a little under the weather. This immunity-boosting version includes ginger, carrots, parsnips, kale, and bone broth.

Ingredients

- 1 tablespoon of avocado oil

- ½ small, finely diced onion

- 2 large carrots (peeled and chopped)

- 1 large parsnip (peeled and chopped)

- 3 stalks of celery (chopped)

- 3 cloves of garlic (minced)

- 1 pound of boneless chicken (in chunky pieces)

- 2 tablespoons fresh parsley

- 1 teaspoon ground turmeric

- ½ teaspoon ground ginger

- ½ teaspoon salt

- 3 cups chicken bone broth (you can also use chicken or vegetable stock)

- ⅔ cup coconut milk

- 1 small head of kale

Method

1. Heat the avocado oil in a large pot and sauté the onions until they turn translucent.

2. Add the carrots, parsnips, celery, and garlic. Continue to sauté until the veggies are soft, but al dente. This usually takes three to five minutes.

3. Add the chicken and let it brown for a few minutes.

4. Add the spices and stir well. Sauté until you can smell the richness of the turmeric.

5. Add the bone broth and coconut milk, cover with a lid, and simmer for up to an hour.

6. Finally, add the chopped kale and stir the pieces in. Keep on low heat until they are soft and wilted.

7. Serve with gluten-free, whole grain bread.

8. You can add even more veggie goodness to this soup if you prefer. Consider broccoli, cauliflower, or bok choy.

9. If you need more fiber, you can also add ⅓ cup of quinoa or a small sweet potato.

Scrumptious Sauerkraut

We spoke about the magic of fermented foods earlier. Here is a quick and easy recipe to make your own yummy probiotics that are brimming with goodness. Sauerkraut lasts a while in the refrigerator and can be served as a side to most lunches and dinners.

Ingredients

- 1 medium cabbage

- 1 tablespoon caraway seeds

- 1 tablespoon sea salt

- 3 tablespoons chopped or grated ginger (optional)

- ⅔ cup grated carrot

Method

1. Remove large outer leaves from the cabbage and set them aside.

2. Core and shred cabbage into fine strips.

3. Mix cabbage strips with caraway seeds, salt, ginger, and carrots.

4. Massage with your hands or mallet for about ten minutes to release the juice.

5. Place into a wide mouth jar and pound down until the juices surface and cover the mixture. Leave about two inches of space at the top.

6. Place whole cabbage leaves on top (inside the jar) and seal the jar firmly. This helps the fermentation process.

7. Keep at room temperature in a dark spot (or cover with a towel) for about three days and then place it in your refrigerator.

8. It can be eaten immediately but improves with time. Enjoy as an accompaniment to any meal, on a sandwich, or have a few mouthfuls on their own as a healthy snack.

No-Bake Tasty Turmeric Bars

These bars are packed with antioxidants and are brilliant anti-inflammatory sweet treats. There's no baking required, and they're gluten, dairy, and refined sugar-free. They're also loaded with healthy fats—no need to feel guilty when enjoying this delicious dessert option.

Turmeric tastes a little bitter on its own, so adding some cinnamon, ginger, and cardamom makes it extra yummy.

Ingredients

Crumbly Crust

- ¾ cup coconut flour

- 1 tablespoon crushed ginger

- 1 tablespoon turmeric

- 1 teaspoon cardamom

- 1 teaspoon cinnamon

- 2 cups almond butter

- ½ cup maple syrup or honey

Flipping Good Filling

- 2 cups sugar-free dark chocolate chips

- ¼ cup coconut oil

- ¼ cup coconut flakes

Method

1. Line a pan with parchment paper and set it aside.

2. Add dry ingredients for the crust to a large bowl, give a good stir, and set aside.

3. Melt almond butter with maple syrup (or honey if you prefer) until combined.

4. Mix the dry and wet ingredients until it forms a thick, smooth batter.

5. Transfer the dough to the lined pan and press firmly. Refrigerate for 30 minutes.

6. Once cooled, melt the chocolate chips and coconut oil and pour over the firm bars.

7. Top with coconut flakes and a dash of cinnamon and turmeric.

8. Freeze until firm and cut into slices.

9. They can be stored in the refrigerator in an airtight container for up to five days.

10. Serve with the golden milk recipe in the next chapter!

Black Bean Brownies

These babies not only taste amazing but they're packed with protein too. I saved it for last because it's my favorite recipe by far! They taste like fudge without the guilt.

Ingredients

- 1 can of black beans (15.5 ounces) - drained and rinsed

- 1 and ½ cups of coconut milk

- 2 tablespoons ground flaxseed (hello omega-3!)

- 6 tablespoons cold water

- ½ cup coconut sugar

- ⅓ cup cacao powder (not cocoa)

- 1 teaspoon kosher salt

- 1 teaspoon baking powder

- ¼ cup dark chocolate chips (plus a few more for the topping)

Method

1. Mix black beans with coconut milk and place them in the refrigerator for eight hours, or ideally overnight. This is the secret step that takes out the 'beany' flavor.

2. Strain beans from the coconut milk and rinse.

3. Preheat the oven to 350 degrees Fahrenheit.

4. Mix the flaxseed and cold water in a small cup and allow it to sit for 10 minutes. They will gel together to form a "flax egg."

5. Combine the beans, flax egg, and coconut sugar in a blender. Pulse until smooth.

6. Add cacao powder, baking powder, and salt. Pulse until smooth again.

7. Add dark chocolate chips and pulse a couple of times - just until the chips have broken slightly.

8. Transfer the brownie mixture to a baking dish and spread evenly.

9. Sprinkle additional chocolate chips on each brownie.

10. Bake at 350 degrees Fahrenheit for eight to 10 minutes or until the crust is firm (the insides should still be soft).

11. Garnish with salt to taste and slice into pieces.

Sometimes you simply want an easy alternative and something that is quick to prepare but still holding loads of nutritious goodness. That is why I included the next chapter that includes recipes for simple and delicious anti-inflammatory drinks.

8

10 ANTI-INFLAMMATORY DRINKS

If your digestive system is particularly sensitive, or if you have trouble getting all your greens in, then juices and smoothies can go a long way to fill up on anti-inflammatory nutrients. They are high in vitamins, minerals, and antioxidants but can be blended in a jiffy and drunk on the way to work. These drink recipes offer a wealth of free-radical-fighting compounds that fight inflammation, provide a healthy dose of vitamins and minerals, and support your overall wellness. Give your immune system a boost with one of these every day.

Astonishing Apple Carrot Beet Smoothie

This goodie smoothie is packed with antioxidants and is a delicious combination of beets, ginger, carrots, orange, and apple. Now you can literally drink your veggies. It's low in calories but high in inflammatory fighting ingredients, and raw beets are earthy and sweet.

Ingredients

- 1 medium red beet, cut into 2-inch chunks

- 1 apple, any variety, cut into 2-inch chunks

- 3 carrots, ends trimmed, cut into 2-inch chunks

- 1 orange (juiced)

- 1 two-inch piece of peeled, fresh ginger

- 1 cup cold water

Method

1. Place all the ingredients in a high-powered blender.

2. Blend until smooth (approximately two minutes).

3. Pour into glasses and enjoy straight away or chill in the refrigerator.

Bonus Tips

- Red beets add a sweet flavor and rich red color, but you can also use yellow beets for a golden-colored smoothie.

- Granny Smith apples give this drink a sour zing, but you can go with any variety.

- Carrots give this one a good kick of fiber.

- Anti-inflammatory ginger adds some heat and spice.

- Orange juice adds that extra, natural sweetness. You can also use coconut water if you prefer.

- Leave the peel on the veggies and fruit for extra fiber and texture. It makes the smoothie thicker and more filling.

- Ginger should, however, be peeled because it can be rather rough and difficult to digest.

- Boost your smoothies with superfoods. You can always add turmeric, chia seeds, cinnamon, or maca powder. This revs up the nutrition.

- Before cutting the red beet, place a sheet of parchment paper on your cutting board to prevent staining.

- If you allow the smoothie to rest, it will separate. Just give a good shake or stir before serving.

Pineapple Tropical Turmeric Smoothie

By now, you'll know that turmeric is a miracle spice that tames inflammation. Tropical fruits add a delightful sweetness and immunity boost to the mixture. It's creamy and delicious.

Ingredients

- 1 cup dairy-free milk

- 2 cups frozen pineapple chunks

- 1 banana

- 1 tablespoon fresh turmeric (or 1 teaspoon ground turmeric)

- 1 teaspoon fresh ginger (or 1/3 teaspoon ground ginger)

Method

1. Add all the ingredients to a blender.

2. Blend for 30 seconds on high or until creamy.

3. Serve chilled (add a slice of pineapple and a paper umbrella if you're at a barbecue - not even kidding)

Bonus Tips

- You only need a small amount of turmeric to get results. Try not to add too much more than the recipe suggests - this can leave a strong aftertaste.

- Turmeric comes in fresh and dried form. Usually, one is good for cooking and the other for blended drinks, but it also depends on how much punch you want in your smoothie!

- Raw turmeric roots look a lot like ginger. The orange flesh is bitter and a little peppery. It's more pungent than dried turmeric. When you buy them at the market, always go for firm roots (soft and shriveled is a no-go).

- You can slice, cube, or grate the roots.

- 1-inch of fresh turmeric = 1 tablespoon grated turmeric = 1 teaspoon ground turmeric

- Ground, dried turmeric loses some pungency and retains its strong color—the stronger the aroma, the better the quality.

- Use frozen pineapple for a thicker consistency, but opt for fresh bananas.

- Ideally, the milk should be non-dairy. Choose almond, cashew, or oat milk.

Green Juice with Gumption

Making green juice can be different every day. It's refreshing and healthy, and you can literally toss in any of your favorite greens! Here are the ingredients we chose: Kale because it adds a beautiful emerald color and offers a healthy, grassy flavor. Celery gives fiber and slight saltiness. Cucumber is mild, low in calories, and provides most of the liquid. Ginger adds spice, lime gives some tart, and apple balanced with sweetness.

Ingredients

- 1 cucumber, sliced

- 3 stalks celery, sliced

- 3 leaves kale, removed from stem

- 1 cup spinach (baby leaves)

- 1-piece fresh ginger (approximately a 1–2-inch chunk)

- 2 tablespoons lime juice

- 2 apples, cored and sliced

Method

1. Place cucumber and celery into a high-powered blender and blend until smooth.

2. Add the remaining ingredients and blend for about two minutes or until smooth.

97

3. Pour the juice through a fine-mesh strainer (or, alternatively, a nut-milk bag).

4. Discard the solid bits.

5. Chill and serve.

Bonus Tips

- The only real difference between a green smoothie and green juice is that you strain the juice. This is helpful if you battle to digest fiber.

- The juice tastes best right after straining, but it can stay in the refrigerator overnight too.

- The juice may turn a little brown after a few hours due to the apples oxidizing. But it's still fine to drink.

- Feel free to customize your juice. Add lots of greens - try some lettuce or broccoli!

- Keep sugar levels down by using healthy liquid bases such as celery, cucumber, or coconut water. Fruit juices should be used sparingly.

- Add some herbs like parsley, basil, and cilantro. It adds an interesting herbal note.

- Remember to boost with superfoods!

Tasty Turmeric Tea

Turmeric tea is a warm and soothing brew that will fight inflammation while tasting good at the same time. It's a rich blend of turmeric, lemon juice, and honey. This recipe also has a pinch of ground black pepper, which helps your body absorb the curcumin (that's the powerful antioxidant found in turmeric). You can drink this right before bedtime.

Ingredients

- 1/2 teaspoon ground turmeric

- 1/4 teaspoon black pepper

- 2 tablespoons lemon juice

- 2 cups water

- 2 teaspoons raw honey

Method

1. Add water, turmeric, lemon juice, and black pepper to a small pot.

2. Whisk together and boil over high heat.

3. Once it starts to boil, turn the heat down and allow it to simmer for 10 minutes.

4. After simmering, add honey and allow the tea to cool for about a minute.

5. Pour into a mug through a strainer to remove the pepper.

6. Serve with slices of lemon, and enjoy!

Bonus Tips

- Have some fun and customize your tea! Add a sprinkle of cinnamon or make it richer with a bag of chamomile tea as it simmers.

- In cold winter months, add a cinnamon stick. It gives a lovely toasty flavor.

- You can also swap the lemon juice for orange juice and a pinch of cloves.

- Trade the honey for maple syrup if you want extra sweetness.

- Add a dash of nutmeg for some zing!

Gorgeous Ginger Shots

Anti-inflammatory ginger shots are intensely flavored little powerhouses. They're a super-concentrated burst of ginger. They're great for your digestion, boost your immune system, and are high in antioxidants.

Ingredients

- 1/4 cup ginger root, washed and roughly chopped

- 1/3 cup lemon juice, from three to four lemons

- 1/4 cup coconut water

- Pinch of cayenne pepper

Method

1. Wash and chop the ginger root. No need to peel because you'll be straining it before serving.

2. Juice the lemons (talk about some powerful vitamin C right there!)

3. Pop all the ingredients into a blender and blend until smooth (no chunks of ginger remaining).

4. Strain well. Press well to ensure you get all the juice out.

5. Serve in shot glasses and enjoy.

Bonus Tips

- Ginger is related to turmeric, cardamom, and galangal. It's been used to treat nausea, indigestion, muscle soreness, and osteoarthritis. It also helps to lower blood sugar, improve brain function, and prevent heart disease. Bottoms up, I say!

- Ginger root tastes spicy when raw, but the ginger powder is more earthy.

- Fresh ginger gives a fiery burn on your tongue when downing shots. Follow with a glass of water if it's too intense for you.

- Don't drink more than one shot a day - too much ginger can cause heartburn.

- Add even more health benefits by adding raw honey, turmeric, aloe vera juice, or apple cider vinegar.

- Double up on the recipe if you want a shot each day. They stay fresh for about a week in the refrigerator (in a sealed container).

Golden Sunset Milk

Golden, turmeric milk is a blend of anti-inflammatory spice and dairy-free milk along with a dash of pepper, cinnamon, and maple syrup. This one packs a real punch for autoimmune disorders.

Dairy-free milk choices include cashew, almond, coconut, or oat milk.

Ayurvedic and Chinese medicine have been prescribing this tonic for centuries. It's soothing just before bedtime and promotes a good night's sleep.

Ingredients

- 2 cups non-dairy milk

- 1 teaspoon ground turmeric

- Pinch of black pepper

- 1/4 teaspoon ground cinnamon

- 1-2 tablespoons maple syrup

- Optional:

  - 1/2 tablespoon coconut oil

  - ginger

  - cardamom

  - peppercorns

    ○   vanilla extract or vanilla bean

Method

1. Pour milk into a small pot on medium heat.

2. Add turmeric, a pinch of pepper, cinnamon, and maple syrup.

3. Bring to a simmer for 10 minutes, allowing all the flavors to merge together.

4. Serve and enjoy.

Bonus Tips

- If you're using nut milk, add some coconut oil. If you're using coconut milk, it has enough of its own fat. This fatty extra helps your body absorb the other ingredients.

- Coconut oil also helps the turmeric milk treat froth a little.

- Sprinkle cinnamon and vanilla bean on the top for some extra decadence.

Jamu Juice

This is a traditional Indonesian herbal drink. It's a simple blend of turmeric, ginger, lemon, and honey. You can serve it warm or chilled, and you'll feel the effects soon after. It is a powerful concoction!

Ingredients

- 125 grams fresh turmeric (approximately 1 cup, roughly chopped)

- 20 grams fresh ginger (approximately 1 finger-sized piece)

- 4 cups coconut water

- 1 lemon, juiced

- 2 tablespoons honey

- Pinch of black pepper (optional)

Method

1. Slice the turmeric and ginger into thin pieces. You can peel them or leave the skin on - up to you.

2. Add the turmeric, ginger, black pepper, and water to a high-speed blender.

3. Blend for about one minute until it's completely smooth.

4. Pour into a pot and bring to a boil.

5. Allow simmering for about 20 minutes.

6. After simmering, add the lemon juice and honey.

7. Give it all a good stir.

8. Strain through a fine-mesh sieve or nut milk bag.

9. Pour into a glass bottle and refrigerate.

Bonus Tips

- Rinse and clean the spicy roots.

- Turmeric can stain your clothes and surfaces. Wash your blender and chopping board as soon as you are done.

- You can use regular water instead of coconut water if you prefer it less rich.

- This is great in the mornings to prime your digestion. Don't down this during a meal, though. It has a very strong, sometimes overpowering flavor.

Golden Beet and Spicy Carrot Juice

This is a vision-boosting, gut-healing wonder of juices! It's packed with beta carotene and powerful nutrients.

Ingredients

- 2 golden beets, chopped

- 1 large carrot, chopped

- 1 banana (peeled, sliced, and frozen)

- 4 mandarin oranges, peeled

- 1 lemon, juiced

- 1/4 teaspoon turmeric powder

- 1 1/2 cup cold water

- Optional topping:

    - grated carrot

    - hemp seeds

Method

1. Add all the ingredients into a high-powered blender.

2. Blend until smooth.

3. Pour into glasses and add your toppings. Voila!

Bonus Tips

- Golden beets' color gives them away. They're full of nutrients (such as beta carotene) that are brilliant for your eyesight.

- Carrots are also vision kings - what a powerful combination!

Elderberry Elixir Tea

This warm and comforting tea wards off colds and flu. The purple berries are packed with vitamins, minerals, and immune-boosting goodies.

Elderberries are often used in cold and flu treatments like cold capsules, lozenges, and syrups. This tea comes without the added sugar and thickeners. Drink it whenever you feel run down or like your immune system needs a boost.

Ingredients

- 2 cups water

- 2 tablespoons dried elderberries

- 1 cinnamon stick

  (yes… it's that simple!)

Method

1. Add water, dried elderberries, and cinnamon stick to a saucepan.

2. Stir well on high heat, bringing the mixture to a boil.

3. Allow simmering for 15 minutes.

4. Let the tea cool after simmering (for about five minutes).

5. Strain through a fine-mesh strainer into a mug.

6. Sip and enjoy!

Bonus Tips

- Elderberries contain antioxidants that boost the immune system. They have been used for centuries to fight respiratory infections.

- They're high in flavonoids, vitamin A, vitamin C, and dietary fiber.

- They're well known for reducing inflammation and providing pain relief.

- Anthocyanin is responsible for these benefits, in addition to the deep purple color.

- Elderberries have a mild flavor, so you can get creative with juices, herbs, and spices. Good additions include ginger, turmeric, lemon, orange slices, and rosemary sprigs.

- You can swap some of the water with cherry juice (unsweetened) for an extra punch of antioxidants.

- Add even more cinnamon if you're struggling with your blood sugar levels.

- Dried hibiscus flowers deepen the ruby red color and help lower blood pressure.

- Add raw honey or maple syrup for a dash of sweetness.

- The elderberries become darker red the longer you boil them. If you prefer a lighter-colored tea, simply reduce the time on the stove.

- Chill the brew in the refrigerator to serve a delicious iced tea (with ice cubes and a sprig of rosemary).

Blissful Blueberry Smoothie

Once again, I've left the best recipe for last. This smoothie is creamy, sweet, and delicious. In addition, it's jam-packed with vitamins, nutrients, and antioxidants. It also doubles up as a refreshing breakfast.

Ingredients

- 2 cups coconut water

- 2 cups frozen blueberries

- 1 frozen banana

- 1/2 cup greek yogurt (or dairy-free coconut yogurt)

- 1 tablespoon flax seeds

Method

1. Throw all the ingredients into a high-powered blender.

2. Blend for about 30 seconds until you have a thick, smooth, and luscious smoothie.

3. Serve in tall glasses and garnish with berries.

Bonus Tips

- For a thinner, less chilled smoothie, use fresh blueberries and bananas instead of frozen ones.

- Blueberries are loaded with phytonutrients that help fight cancer, lower blood pressure, and improve your cardiovascular health.

- Bananas are known for their potassium punch and a solid dose of magnesium. These support heart and digestive health and are also excellent anti-inflammatories.

- Coconut water is loaded with electrolytes, vitamins, and minerals.

- Flax seeds are great little shots of Omega-3 fatty acids and fiber. They also thicken the smoothie beautifully.

9

THE ANTI-INFLAMMATORY
LIFESTYLE

Tackling inflammation in our bodies isn't just about food and dietary choices. Other contributing factors include sleep, stress, menopause, antibiotics, and pollution. We'll look at these more closely in this chapter.

The Importance of Sleep

Losing sleep or having interrupted sleep (even for part of a single night) can trigger the key cellular pathway that produces inflammation. The connection between sleep and inflammation is rooted in the microbiome in our gut.

The world of microorganisms in our digestive tract is often referred to as our "second brain" (Gulbin, 2020). It's home to an entire nervous system of its own, with over 100 million neurons. This web of signals is in constant communication with our brain. This helps to regulate our hormones, appetite, digestion, metabolism, mood, and stress levels.

The microbiome produces and releases sleep-influencing neurotransmitters, including melatonin, dopamine, serotonin, and gamma-aminobutyric acid (GABA).

These millions of bacteria in our gut are regulated by circadian rhythms. When these are thrown out of whack, the microbiome responds. Not getting enough sleep affects this delicate balance, quite literally, overnight.

Research shows that insomnia leads to a significant decrease in beneficial bacteria, an increase in insulin sensitivity, and it also exacerbates symptoms associated with obesity and types 2 diabetes (Michael, 2016). There is also an undeniable connection between better quality of sleep and higher levels of beneficial gut microbes.

The hormone melatonin is essential to sleep and a healthy sleep-wake cycle. It also contributes to maintaining gut health. Melatonin deficiency has been linked to leaky gut syndrome (increased permeability of the gastrointestinal tract). Melatonin is produced in the gut and brain, and generation of the intestinal type operates on a different circadian rhythm.

Another critical hormone to the sleep-wake cycle is cortisol. Cortisol levels usually rise early in the day and promote alertness, focus, and energy. The balance of this hormone is a delicate one, and it is one of the first responders to stress (increasing the inflammatory response) and directly affects gut permeability. When this balance is disturbed, we may have trouble falling asleep and wake up groggy.

Disruptions to circadian rhythms upset the microbial rhythms. This can happen with irregular bedtimes, jet lag, and shift work. Changes to microbial rhythms can result in metabolic imbalance, glucose intolerance, and weight gain.

Stress is one of the main disruptors of our sleep. Recent research in Japan revealed that students who took probiotics eight weeks before an exam slept better than the placebo group. Despite high levels of stress, students on a probiotic supplement experienced less difficulty falling asleep, maintained their deep, slow-wave sleep, and woke to feel rested (Breus, 2019).

Stress and Inflammation

When you're psychologically stressed, your body goes into the "fight or flight" response. This releases the stress hormone, cortisol, which suppresses your immune response and digestion. Cortisol also fuels the production of glucose, inhibits insulin production, and narrows the arteries. This forces your blood to pump harder.

Stress also releases the hormone, adrenaline. This sends a message to your body to increase the heart and respiratory rate, which expands your airways to send more oxygen to your muscles.

In addition, stress decreases lymphocytes (white blood cells) which are an essential part of your immune system, which puts you at greater risk for viruses like the common cold.

A chronic state of stress can lead to multiple inflammatory responses. Cytokines are kicked up a notch, and the cycle of stress and inflammation becomes your body's "new normal."

Taking steps to alleviate stress will go a long way in helping to stabilize your body's immune response. This can include exercise, meditation, and mindfulness techniques.

Menopause and Inflammation

The hormones estrogen and progesterone have an important and complex effect on the body's inflammatory response. Both of these hormones decline during perimenopause and menopause, and both usually have an anti-inflammatory effect on the body. This decrease removes the natural protection against inflammation, and this is why women often experience inflammatory symptoms such as body aches and pains.

One of the best tips for women at this life stage is to take an evening primrose oil supplement. It helps balance your hormones, minimizes hormonal acne and hair loss, and eases joint pain.

The Terrible Downside of Antibiotics

Antibiotics are designed to kill bacteria that make us sick. Unfortunately, it also kills the good bacteria in our gut. Some of the flora never get the chance to grow back and multiply, which weakens the microbiome environment considerably. This is why it's essential to take probiotic supplements when on a course of antibiotics.

A recent Danish study discovered a three-fold increase in inflammatory bowel disease in children who received more than seven courses of antibiotics (Groth, 2011).

Pollution and Other Environmental Factors

We live in a world that is filled with industrial chemicals and pollutants. We all have xenobiotics (substances foreign to our body) lurking around inside us. Although we can't eliminate all of what we're exposed to, there are ways we can decrease the burden on our bodies.

This isn't just about avoiding fumes and giving up smoking. Chemicals are well hidden in many of our cleaning and beauty products, medicine, and cooking aids.

We will always have a degree of toxic exposure. We need to wash our hair, put on make-up, clean our homes, and keep pests away. Our lives are made easier by nonstick cookware and water in plastic bottles.

The way we can lower our exposure is to choose natural, botanical products and non-toxic cleaners. Go slow on air freshener and hard-core sanitizing chemicals. Try to cut back on over-the-counter medications such as ibuprofen, allergy remedies, and acid blockers. You may find that as you shift your diet to anti-inflammatory foods, you may need less and less of these anyway.

Not only can you purchase natural products for your home and body, but you can also even make some of them at home yourself. For example, simple coconut oil is often used in skincare, moisturizers, and hair conditioners. Look for natural beauty products and make-up that are gluten-free and contain natural plant-based ingredients.

You can clean your home with vinegar water spray, scrub with baking soda, combine rubbing alcohol and water to clean mirrors and windows, and olive oil is fantastic for polishing wood surfaces.

Try to keep houseplants in your home. They naturally clean the air and look great too! If you have pets, you may wish to invest in an air cleaner in your bedroom and office area. Avoid chemical air fresheners and opt for essential oil diffusers as a less harmful way to keep your home fresh and smelling good.

Keep fresh air and ventilation going by opening the

windows, and decorate your home with natural materials such as bamboo, stone, wool, wood, and organic cotton. Test your home for mold and use a proper filter in your vacuum cleaner.

Natural products can also be used outside. Lawn care and pest control companies now have many environmentally friendly and non-toxic products.

Medications take a real toll on your liver because it needs to process and eliminate the toxins. Some prescriptions may be essential for some conditions, but there are some minor ailments that can be solved with natural remedies instead of popping a pill. For example, if you have a headache or menstrual cramps, try some turmeric instead of ibuprofen. Turmeric is a powerful anti-inflammatory and decreases swelling, which is often the cause of the pain. You can even buy it in capsule form in addition to sprinkling it over your food. If you're struggling with heartburn or reflux, sip on some raw apple cider vinegar. It's a much healthier choice than chewing on an antacid. A spoonful of this tart liquid might make you cringe, but you'll be surprised at how effective it is.

Of course, many of these choices come down to your personal lifestyle, what is aggravating inflammation in your unique body's constitution, and what will work for you in the long term.

In the next chapter, we'll take a look at the inflammation spectrum, how you can find your specific place on it, and how to restore your unique balance.

10

THE INFLAMMATION SPECTRUM

Although we're all similar in basic biology, we each have very unique biochemistry. Each individual has a specific combination and interconnection of genetics, lifestyle, environment, hormone fluctuations, and microbiome habitat.

What causes inflammation in your body might be the complete opposite of someone else. The precise effect of inflammation on your body is also highly unique. One person expresses chronic inflammation on their skin. Others suffer from stomach cramps and insomnia.

In addition, you're constantly changing. Your symptoms may change in subtle ways, and your reaction to one food type now may be different in a few years.

Your body falls on the inflammation spectrum in a very

unique spot, and it's important to figure out what works and doesn't work for your body. Your lifestyle and dietary choices will either increase or decrease inflammation, and this bio-individuality can be determined through a process of elimination. Your diet needs to work optimally for you. Although this book gives you a general idea of what foods to include and exclude, the subtle shifts are left for you to discover. What is medicine for one person is another person's inflammatory trigger.

Through trial and error, you'll be able to figure out your specific intolerances and sensitivities. You may even be eating something on a daily basis that is contributing to major inflammation that you're unaware of. Even a healthy, anti-inflammatory food type may aggravate your symptoms.

The following questions will help you determine how your body uniquely reacts to inflammation. Tick each one that applies to you:

Brain and Nervous System

- Do you struggle with memory loss or find that you are more absent-minded than usual? For example, losing things or missing appointments.

- Are you sad, depressed, or irritable for no obvious reason?

- Are you anxious and panicky?

- Do you have difficulty concentrating or focusing?

- Do you have unexplained mood swings?

- Are you having sensory issues, such as experiencing sound or smell differently than you once did?

- Does your family have a history of dementia or Alzheimer's disease?

Digestive System

- Are you often bloated, or is your stomach distended after or between meals?

- Do you struggle with diarrhea or loose stool?

- Are you often constipated?

- Are your stools hard and small, like tiny pellets?

- Do you get acid reflux or heartburn after eating?

- Do you have issues with bad breath?

- Is your stomach distended after eating certain foods?

- Do you often have abdominal cramps and bloating?

- Are you occasionally nauseous after eating?

- Does your stomach respond when you're anxious or stressed (gas, bloating, diarrhea)?

Detoxification System

- Do you retain water easily?

- If you press your finger into your arm or leg, does it leave a pit for a few seconds?

- Does your weight go up and down during the day (fluctuating by more than five pounds)?

- Have you been diagnosed with chronic infections such as Lyme disease?

- Do you have a yellowish tint to your skin or whites of your eyes?

- Is your abdomen tender, especially in the upper right quadrant?

- Is your urine dark yellow and pungent?

- Is your skin itchy, flaking, or covered in a rash?

Insulin System

- Do you often crave sweets and starchy foods?

- Has your appetite increased or decreased?

- Are you more thirsty than normal?

- Do you urinate more often?

- Have you noticed your vision blurring occasionally?

- Are you very fatigued despite getting enough sleep?

- Is your tiredness alleviated if you eat something?

- Do you feel light-headed, dizzy, or shaky if you don't eat for a few hours?

- Are you irritable if you skip a meal?

- Is your waist wider than your hips?

- Do you struggle to lose weight even when you eat less?

- Do you have high blood sugar?

Hormonal (Endocrine) System

- Are you tired in the afternoons and get a second wind at night?

- Do you get regular headaches or migraines?

- Are you dizzy if you stand up too quickly?

- Do you crave salty foods?

- Do your hands and feet get cold easily?

- Do you tend to sleep too much?

- Are the outer thirds of your eyebrows thinning or missing entirely?

- Has your sex drive diminished?

- Women: Do you have irregular, painful, or unusually heavy periods?

- Men: Do you suffer from erectile dysfunction?

Musculoskeletal System

- Do your joints hurt? This could be periodic pain, a constant ache, or random flares with the pain coming and going.

- Are you hypermobile, hyper-flexible, or double-jointed?

- Are you prone to accidents, such as twisting your ankle, tripping, falling, or dropping things? Do you feel clumsy? Are your tendons and ligaments often torn or stretched?

- Do your joints pop, crack, snap, or get stuck?

- Do you wake up in the mornings with stiff and achy joints or muscles? Is this initially alleviated with movement, only to return hours later?

- Do you suffer from constant neck and back pain, tightness, or tension?

- Do you often get "pins and needles?"

- Do you experience random stabbing pains or numbness in your hands and feet?

- Do you have shooting pains, especially down your arms and legs?

- Do you find massages painful, especially in your limbs and buttocks area?

Autoimmune Inflammation

- Do you experience extreme reactions to particular foods or after eating? This can be things such as vomiting, diarrhea, pain, skin reactions, or neurological episodes (brain fog or panic attacks, for example).

- Are you intolerant to cold or heat?

- Do your hands and feet turn blue or gray when you are cold?

- Are your skin, mouth, or eyes especially dry?

- Does your family have a history of autoimmune issues? These can include rheumatoid arthritis, lupus, multiple sclerosis, celiac disease, inflammatory bowel disease, Crohn's disease, or Hashimoto's thyroiditis.

- Do you suffer from painful and swollen joints?

- Do you experience bilateral numbness and tingling (in the same place on both sides of your body - for example, both elbows or both feet)

- Do you suffer from rashes, chronic acne, recurring boils, or cystic acne? This can be on your face or body.

- Do you suffer from extreme and constant fatigue that isn't relieved by sleeping, eating, or other remedies (for example, meditation, yoga, relaxation techniques)?

Your Unique Profile

After answering these questions, do you notice one or more specific parts of your system that are responding adversely to inflammation? Are you struggling more with musculoskeletal symptoms or more with your nervous system?

Here are specific dietary tips for each system that you can use to target your unique immune response:

Brain and Nervous System

Inflammation of the brain and nervous system results in brain fog, problems concentrating, mood swings, depression, and memory trouble. In the long-term, it can lead to cognitive impairment, dementia, and Alzheimer's.

Just like some people struggle with the leaky gut syndrome, a similar thing can happen in our brains with the blood-brain barrier. Bacterial toxins released into the bloodstream can trigger an inflammatory response.

There are specific foods and supplements that will help you decrease inflammation in your brain. After just a few days, you may notice an improvement in your mood and concentration.

Try to incorporate the following into your diet:

- Wild-caught fish (ideally fatty fish like salmon). Omega-3 fatty acids are brain-boosting miracles.

- Medium-chain triglyceride (MCT) oil (extracted from coconut and palm oil) improves cognitive function, focus, and concentration.

- Lion's mane mushrooms. They contain nerve growth factors that help to regenerate and protect brain tissue.

- Mucuna pruriens (also called kapikacchu) is an Ayurvedic herb that helps the body adapt to stress. It's rich in levodopa (L-dopa), the precursor to dopamine (the feel-good hormone).

- Krill oil supplements. This contains 50 times more of the antioxidant astaxanthin than most fish oil supplements. Krill oil contains phospholipids that support brain and nerve function.

- Magnesium enhances learning and memory, increases neuroplasticity, and supports various brain receptors. Deficiencies often lead to anxiety, depression, attention deficit hyperactivity disorder (ADHD), brain fog, and headaches. High doses are found in supplement form, and the following foods are also rich in magnesium: pumpkin seeds, almonds, spinach, cashews, and avocados.

- Cardiovascular exercise improves the product of brain-derived neurotrophic factor (BDNF), boosts memory, and makes you feel better emotionally. BDNF helps the growth and healthy functioning of nerves.

- Valerian root helps to modulate the neurotransmitter GABA. Healthy GABA levels increase BDNF levels, and can improve symptoms of impaired memory, and lowers the risk of Alzheimer's disease.

Digestive System

Gut dysfunction is the most common ailment when it comes to inflammation. This includes constipation, diarrhea, irritable bowel syndrome (IBS), small intestinal bacterial overgrowth (SIBO), bloating, and acid reflux. There is also the likelihood of esophageal damage, stomach ulcers, and leaky gut syndrome.

Calming inflammation in your gut can have a positive ripple effect throughout your system.

Here are some foods and supplements that decrease inflammation in your digestive tract:

- Eat cooked vegetables instead of raw as this makes them easier to digest. Try to steam them instead of boiling (the latter removes much of the nutritional value). You can puree them in a blender or make a hearty soup to make them even more digestible.

- Bone broth. Be careful not to overcook the broth, as extended cooking times can result in inflammatory histamines being released. Galangal broth, made from the galangal root (closely related to ginger), is suitable for vegans. Both types are anti-inflammatory and have a soothing, healing effect on the gut. They make an excellent soup base.

- Fermented vegetables and drinks such as sauerkraut, kefir, and kombucha. The beneficial bacteria support gastrointestinal happiness.

- Probiotic supplements improve the balance of bacteria, and it's a good idea to change them up every few months. This promotes microbiome variety. Remember to always take these if you're ever on antibiotics.

- Glutamine supplements are amino acids that target the healing of the gut lining.

- Digestive enzymes (betaine HCL with pepsin). This helps your body digest protein and fat more easily.

- Licorice root is a soothing and healing supplement for your intestine lining, especially if you suffer from the leaky gut syndrome.

- Slippery elm powder is a miracle remedy for irritable bowel syndrome. It calms down cramping, bloating, and gas. It's also great for the bowel lining.

Detoxification System

Your detoxification system includes your liver, lymphatic

system, kidneys, and gallbladder. They process and remove toxins such as alcohol, drugs, pesticides, pollutants, and metabolic waste products.

If inflammation strikes your detox system, waste can start to build up in your body, and this causes further inflammation. You may be prone to lymphatic backup, fatty liver disease, gallbladder problems, or a general feeling of malaise.

This system also applies to Lyme disease, mold exposure, severe alcohol or drug use, or people who need to take daily prescription medication.

You can calm down the inflammation and promote your body's natural detoxification by having more of the following:

- Dandelion tea is a natural liver tonic and contains B vitamins. These are essential for detoxification.

- Spirulina powder or supplements. This green goodness is powerful when it comes to getting rid of waste products.

- Red clover blossom tea (also available in powder or supplement form). A strong liver fan, this tea helps the detoxification organ do its job more efficiently.

- Milk thistle tea. Also targeted to the liver, this tea helps decrease heavy metal damage (which often comes from polluted environments).

- Parsley and cilantro also get to work on heavy metals, including lead and mercury. They are easy herbs to add to any main meal.

- Veggies that contain sulfur, such as garlic, onion, Brussels sprouts, cabbage, cauliflower, and broccoli.

They help your liver break down toxins effectively. Broccoli sprouts are even more potent than normal broccoli because they contain sulforaphane which supports detox pathways.

- Leafy greens. You can't have too many of these! As we said earlier in the book, the darker, the better. You can reach for kale, spinach, and chard. These greens contain folate, which opens detoxification pathways. Liver function can be supported by eating bitter greens, too (such as collard greens, mustard greens, and arugula).

- Dry brush your skin before showering. Your skin is an organ and one of the primary ways your body gets rid of toxins. Brush up your legs and arms towards your torso, and then brush your torso outwards toward the armpits and groin. This follows the path of the lymph nodes. If you dry brush every day, you'll support your lymphatic system by moving excess fluid and lymph from the body. This includes the waste they are carrying. You'll decrease the 'puffy' look of your skin, which is caused by sluggish lymph.

Blood Sugar System

When your blood sugar spikes too often, you're put at risk for insulin resistance. This can take many forms: metabolic syndrome, prediabetes, obesity, and type 2 diabetes. Further complications of diabetes include nerve pain, cardiovascular disease, kidney damage, and vision impairment.

An imbalance in the blood sugar and insulin system is often due to inflammation in the liver and overworked cellular insulin receptors. They lose their sensitivity to insulin's sugar-balancing effects.

To tame this inflammatory fire, you need to add at least some of the following to your diet and lifestyle:

- Cinnamon. You can add this to tea, warm drinks, fruit salad, oats, and various other foods. Cinnamon contains proanthocyanidins, and these change insulin signals in fat cells (in a good way). It reduces blood sugar levels and triglycerides in people with type 2 diabetes.

- Reishi mushrooms are medicinal and help lower blood sugar levels. They do this by downregulating alpha-glucosidase, which is the enzyme that breaks down starches into sugars. Reishi mushrooms are available as tea, powder, or in dried form.

- Berberine supplements. This is a plant-based alkaloid widely used in Chinese medicine. It delays the breakdown of carbs into sugars. This helps to regulate blood sugar levels and can be as powerful as metformin for keeping blood sugar balanced in people with diabetes.

- Matcha green tea. Matcha contains epigallocatechin gallate (EGCG), which helps to stabilize blood sugar levels. The powdered form is particularly powerful because it contains the whole green tea leaf.

- Apple cider vinegar improves insulin sensitivity and the way your system responds to sugar. It also promotes lower fasting blood sugar levels.

- Vegetables that are high in fiber. Whole-food plant sources of fiber are effective at improving insulin sensitivity and lowering glucose metabolism. Some real gems include artichokes, broccoli, Brussels sprouts, carrots, turnips, and beets.

- D-chiro-inositol supplements play an integral part in insulin signaling and also decrease insulin resistance.

- Chromium supplements are minerals that affect insulin-signaling pathways. It improves insulin sensitivity and also lowers triglyceride and cholesterol levels.

Hormone (Endocrine) System

Hormones that are imbalanced can wreak all sorts of havoc on your body and emotions. You may suffer from moodiness, PMS, painful or irregular menstrual cycles, and low sex drive. Women in perimenopause or going through menopause have a particularly hard time trying to rebalance.

There are other ways your hormonal system lets you know that things are out of balance. These can include issues with your thyroid, adrenal fatigue, or testosterone imbalances.

Whatever your specific hormonal imbalance, including these specific foods and supplements, can help get your system realigned. Reduced inflammation will help improve hormone receptor activity and your brain's communication with the different types of hormones. Even if you're in a hormonal warzone (such as menopause), you will notice improvement with these additions to your diet.

- Sole water. This is electrolyte-infused water that supports the adrenal hormone aldosterone. This plays a role in electrolyte and fluid balance and stabilizes sodium levels. The best part is that you can make it yourself!

- ○ Invest in a large mason jar with a plastic lid (metal lids can oxidize and corrode when exposed to salt)

- ○ Fill it a quarter way up with sea salt (Himalayan pink salt is fantastic too).

- ○ Add filtered water, leaving a bit of room at the top.

- ○ Secure the lid, give it a good shake, and let it sit overnight.

- ○ Check your sole water in the morning. If you see salt at the bottom of the mason jar, the water is saturated. If you don't see any, then add an extra teaspoon.

- ○ Give another good shake and give an hour for it to dissolve properly.

- ○ Continue with this process until there is salt sediment at the bottom.

- ○ When the sole water is completely saturated, it's ready.

- ○ Add one teaspoon of the sole water to a glass of water every morning and drink it before eating anything. Don't use metal utensils (only plastic or wood)

- Sea vegetables. This includes plant foods from the ocean, for example, kelp, nori, dulse, kombu, wakame, and agar. They are rich in iodine which you need to produce thyroid hormones. Every single cell in your body needs these hormones to function optimally.

- Wild-caught, fatty fish (ideally salmon, mackerel, and sardines). They are rich in Omega-3 fatty acids that support hormone balance, as well as vitamin D that is a key player in metabolic pathways.

- Chasteberry supplements. This fancy berry keeps progesterone and estrogen levels in balance.

- Rooibos tea. A bright red tea from an African plant that supports adrenal function. It does this by balancing levels of the stress hormone cortisol.

- Ashwagandha supplements. This herb is the ultimate cortisol balancer. It's popular in Ayurvedic medicine and therapy. Ashwagandha supports the hypothalamic-pituitary-adrenal (HPA) axis and boosts sluggish thyroid hormones. This has a calming effect and helps with mood swings and hormone-fueled anxiety.

- Evening primrose oil supplements. Rich in omega-6 fatty acids, this beneficial oil helps relieve symptoms of menopause, PMS, PCOS, and hormonally-fueled acne.

- Schisandra powder is an adrenal-supporting berry that is easy to add to smoothies and teas.

Musculoskeletal System

Your body is held together by your bones and muscles, and

inflammation of these structures can have many painful effects. This can range from tight and sore muscles and joints to severe cases of osteoarthritis, fibromyalgia, and joint-centered autoimmune diseases (such as rheumatoid arthritis, Sjögren's syndrome, and lupus).

Inflammation in these areas can also compromise the structure of your joints, muscles, and connective tissue. You may be wobbly on your feet and prone to injury or tight with pain and stiffness.

Chronic pain can lead to an inability to exercise, joint damage, and muscle weakness. Incorporating the following foods and supplements will help you move your body more easily and hopefully have much less pain.

- Methylsulfonylmethane (MSM) supplements - MSM contains sulfur which reduces joint and muscle pain by decreasing inflammation.

- Turmeric is an ancient medicinal spice that has been used for centuries as an anti-inflammatory and healing compound.

- Collagen powder is a powder that can be added to smoothies, hot drinks, or cold beverages. It helps heal and restore connective tissue.

- Glucosamine sulfate is a supplement that supports healthy cartilage and soothes synovial fluid between the joints. This reduces pain, improves mobility, and calms inflammation.

- Infrared sauna reduces inflammation, is incredibly relaxing, reduces stress, and relaxes muscles.

- Cryotherapy uses extreme cold for short periods of time to rapidly drive down inflammation. It can result in an instant and significant pain relief.

- Massages - Various techniques such as Swedish, trigger point, myofascial release, and deep-tissue variants will target and relieve muscle pain and tension.

Autoimmunity

Autoimmune diseases are becoming more and more prolific. The immune system destroys body tissues and cells. This can be as severe as a 90 percent destruction of the adrenal glands in Addison's disease - and that's just to be officially diagnosed.

Autoimmune inflammation is brutal, but it happens gradually. Ideally, you're able to start managing the symptoms before they are life-threatening or highly destructive.

Autoimmune diseases generally have three stages of progression:

1. Silent autoimmunity. Antibodies test positive in the lab, but there are no noticeable symptoms yet.

2. Autoimmune reactivity: Once again, the patient is tested positive for antibodies, and they start to experience symptoms.

3. Autoimmune disease (official diagnosis): The body has been destroyed to such an extent that a positive diagnosis can be made, symptoms are more severe, and potential further destruction is anticipated.

When you find yourself somewhere in this spectrum, you may go from doctor to doctor with no definitive answers.

You're not sick enough to be diagnosed, and yet you're still experiencing unexplained and debilitating symptoms.

Inflammation is the primary driver behind most autoimmune diseases. Your immune system thinks your own cells are foreign invaders and mistakes a healthy piece of your body as a clump of bacteria. The most common autoimmune diseases include rheumatoid arthritis, systemic lupus erythematosus, inflammatory bowel disorders, celiac disease, psoriasis, scleroderma, vitiligo, pernicious anemia, Hashimoto's thyroiditis, Addison's disease, Graves' disease, Sjögren's syndrome, type 1 diabetes, hidradenitis supportive, and multiple sclerosis (MS).

These diseases can be mild, or they can be so debilitating that you're bedridden and in constant pain.

Usually, the immune system attacks the digestive system, joints, muscles, skin, connective tissue, brain and spinal cord, endocrine glands (such as the thyroid and adrenals), and blood vessels.

These foods and supplements will tame inflammation and help your body start to restore and rebalance itself.

- Organ meats from grass-fed or pastured animals. Organ meats sound terrible to some, but they contain some of the highest levels of vitamin A, B vitamins, and iron. Autoimmune conditions are often tied to a deficiency in vitamin A.

- Extra-virgin cod-liver oil. This is rich in fat-soluble vitamins, and your immune system needs this type of fat to function properly.

- Emu oil. This is another odd-sounding choice and won't be appealing to vegans for sure, but it's very rich in vitamin K2.

- Broccoli sprouts have some of the highest levels of sulforaphane you can find. This supports methylation, which dramatically reduces inflammation and maintains proper T-cell function (your immune system's SWAT team).

- Elderberry is a fruit that helps balance the immune system. You can find it in liquid supplement form or as a cordial you can add to water.

- Black cumin seed oil. This increases T-regulatory cells and rebalances the immune system.

- Pterostilbene supplements. This acts in a similar way to resveratrol and decreases NF-KB proteins (which are inflammatory), and simultaneously increases nuclear factor erythroid 2 (Nrf2) pathways (which are anti-inflammatory).

- Water or coconut kefir. These are fermented drinks that contain vitamin K2. They also have traces of kefiran that is a unique sugar produced by kefir grains. Kefiran decreases inflammation and calms the immune system.

FINAL WORDS...

This book has a lot of information to take in, and, as you can tell, finding an anti-inflammatory diet and lifestyle that works for you and your specific body type will take time and commitment.

I encourage you to be creative with your eating and to try new things. Jazz up some of your old favorite recipes with some anti-inflammatory zing. Remake your way of cooking and include healthier ingredients in a fun way. Learn new methods, try new products, buy a new pan.

If you're unsure where to start, simply pick one of the simple recipes we included and add your own touch. Get to know your own body and constitution, eliminate and reintroduce, play around with flavors and food groups. Mix and match according to your symptoms and be adventurous with exotic vegetables and spices you may have never tried before. Your culinary horizons can expand and become an adventure all of its own.

If you're worried about falling off the wagon or not being disciplined enough, don't be. Even eating out or going on vacation doesn't have to set you back. Nothing is forbidden. It's all a choice. And, if you do have a bad week, simply pick up and start again. Live your life. Enjoy it.

Feed and nourish yourself in a healthy way most of the time. You don't have to be perfect. You'll soon know that certain foods you're simply better off not eating again. You'll also discover new and wonderful foods that your system loves.

Remember to take this beyond the kitchen. Exercise more - go for that evening walk with your dog. Go to bed earlier and get some proper sleep for a change. Use natural products that feel good on your skin. Treat your body to what it deserves.

You're now equipped to make informed and conscious choices with the food you eat. You may even decide to eat something inflammatory on a special occasion, but because you're aware of how your body will react, perhaps you'll choose to have just a little. You're empowered now. You have control.

As your health improves, you may find that your balanced body can now tolerate a food that it couldn't before. You might find that a slice of birthday cake or a handful of potato chips doesn't send you running to the bathroom anymore. Just keep in mind that too many compromises too often can distract you from listening to your body - and that is the message I want to leave you with:

Pay close attention to your body's feedback. It sends you subtle messages all the time. If you go through a stressful life transition, or if you find yourself in a new phase, such as menopause or pregnancy, pay even more attention.

Listen to your body.

It holds all the answers.

REFERENCES

10+ Anti-Inflammatory Drinks to Boost Your Wellness. (2020, September 13). Downshiftology. https://downshiftology.com/anti-inflammatory-drinks/

Asleep. (n.d.). https://pixabay.com/photos/woman-asleep-girl-sleep-dreams-2197947/

Avocado. (n.d.). https://pixabay.com/photos/avocado-vegetable-food-healthy-2115922/

Berger, M. (2019, August 22). How Intermittent Fasting Can Help Lower Inflammation. Healthline; Healthline Media. https://www.healthline.com/health-news/fasting-can-help-ease-inflammation-in-the-body

Breus, M. (2019, January 2). 5 Things To Know About Sleep And Inflammation. Your Guide to Better Sleep. https://thesleepdoctor.com/2019/01/01/5-things-to-know-about-sleep-and-inflammation/

Breus, M. J. (2016, January 13). How Your Gut Bacteria Informs Your Sleep. HuffPost. https://www.huffpost.com/entry/unlocking-the-sleep-gut-connection_b_8941314?ec_carp=897845873063396954

Bryan, L. (2019, April 3). 8 Anti-Inflammatory Foods I Eat Every Week. Downshiftology. https://downshiftology.com/anti-inflammatory-foods/

Butter. (n.d.). https://pixabay.com/photos/food-butter-table-milk-3179853/

Caporuscio, J. (2019, September 19). Does sugar cause inflammation? What the research says. MedicalNewsToday. https://www.medicalnewstoday.com/articles/326386#reducing-inflammation

Cole, Will. (2021). INFLAMMATION SPECTRUM: find your food triggers and reset your system. Yellow Kite.

E., W. (2019, May 14). The Truth About Meat + Inflammation. Whitney E. RD. https://www.whitneyerd.com/2019/05/the-truth-about-meat-inflammation.html

Finding Balance. (n.d.). https://pixabay.com/photos/yoga-outdoor-woman-pose-young-2176668/

Fritsche, K. L. (2015). The Science of Fatty Acids and Inflammation. Advances in Nutrition, 6(3), 293S301S. https://doi.org/10.3945/an.114.006940

Groth, B. F. de S. (2011, October 10). Help or hindrance? Antibiotics' role in chronic inflammatory diseases. The Conversation. https://theconversation.com/help-or-hindrance-antibiotics-role-in-chronic-inflammatory-diseases-3090

Gulbin, S. (2020, March 24). How Sugar Causes Inflammation in the Body. SpineNation.

https://spinenation.com/wellness/dietnutrition/how
-sugar-causes-inflammation-in-the-body

Human Body. (n.d.).
https://pixabay.com/illustrations/human-skeleton-
human-body-anatomy-163715/

Illness. (n.d.). https://pixabay.com/illustrations/virus-
microscope-infection-illness-1812092/

Immune response: MedlinePlus Medical Encyclopedia.
(2018). MedlinePlus.
https://medlineplus.gov/ency/article/000821.htm

Mainland, S. (2017, April 12). Menopause, Inflammation, and
Joint Pain. Australian Menopause Centre.
https://www.menopausecentre.com.au/information-
centre/articles/menopause-inflammation-and-joint-
pain/

Morris, A., & Rossiter, M. (2011). Anti-Inflammation Diet
For Dummies. John Wiley & Sons.

Pathogen. (n.d.). https://pixabay.com/photos/virus-
pathogen-antibody-antibodies-5741636/

Prasad, A. S. (2014). Zinc: An antioxidant and anti-
inflammatory agent: Role of zinc in degenerative
disorders of aging. Journal of Trace Elements in
Medicine and Biology, 28(4), 364–371.
https://doi.org/10.1016/j.jtemb.2014.07.019

Rath, L. (n.d.). Can Increasing fiber reduce inflammation?
Arthritis Foundation.
https://www.arthritis.org/health-wellness/healthy-

living/nutrition/anti-inflammatory/increasing-
fiber#:~:text=In%20part%2C%20a%20fiber%2Dric
h

Red Meat. (n.d.). https://pixabay.com/photos/meat-food-
bbq-fried-meat-1155132/

Şanlier, N., Gökcen, B. B., & Sezgin, A. C. (2017). Health
benefits of fermented foods. Critical Reviews in Food
Science and Nutrition, 59(3), 506–527.
https://doi.org/10.1080/10408398.2017.1383355

Sauerkraut. (n.d.). https://pixabay.com/photos/carrot-
healthy-fermented-4497968/

Schipani, D. (2018, October 16). The Link Between Stress
and Inflammation. Everyday Health.
https://www.everydayhealth.com/wellness/united-
states-of-stress/link-between-stress-
inflammation/#:~:text=Chronic%20Conditions%20
Linked%20to%20Stress&text=Over%20time%2C%2
0inflammation%20can%20damage

Signs You Have Too Much Inflammation in Your Body.
(2019, December 10). The Apprentice Doctor.
https://www.theapprenticedoctor.com/signs-you-
have-too-much-inflammation-in-your-body/

Simpson, K. (n.d.). The Guide to Naturally Fighting
Inflammation. Dee Cee Laboratories.
https://cdn.chiroeco.com/wp-
content/uploads/2017/05/E-Book_DeeCeeLabs.pdf

Spritzler, F. (2019, December 20). The 13 Most Anti-

Inflammatory Foods You Can Eat. Healthline. https://www.healthline.com/nutrition/13-anti-inflammatory-foods#TOC_TITLE_HDR_12

Stomach. (n.d.). https://pixabay.com/photos/stomach-health-diet-dessert-eating-3532098/

Van De Walle, G. (2020, April 16). Is Dairy Inflammatory? Healthline. https://www.healthline.com/nutrition/is-dairy-inflammatory#dairy

Zelman, D. (2019, October 21). Signs of Chronic Inflammation You May Not Expect. WebMD. https://www.webmd.com/arthritis/ss/slideshow-signs-chronic-inflammation-unexpected

ABOUT THE AUTHOR

I guess I'll say that I'm a gal who has gone against the grain as far back in life as I can remember, but after realizing the nutritional potency and healing power in foods, I've finally decided to start going *with* the grains...yeah, and the vegetables and healthy fruits as well.

I wrote this book to take readers on a health journey with me. As a pharmacist, I have seen just how our food choices just about make or break us. Also, my mother, who always seemed to be a vibrant, jubilant, healthy woman, was diagnosed with and died of cancer at a relatively young age. This event triggered my interest in nutrition as a health resource and served as a wake-up call that we humans can be very fragile. Please enjoy this journey with me and make it your own!

Made in the USA
Columbia, SC
25 May 2021